THE NATURAL WAY SERIES

Increasing numbers of people worldwide are falling victim to illnesses which modern medicine, for all its technical advances, seems often powerless to prevent – and sometimes actually causes. To find cures for these so-called 'diseases of civilization' more and more people are turning to 'natural' medicine for an answer. *The Natural Way* series aims to offer clear, practical and reliable guidance to the safest, gentlest and most effective treatments available – and so to give sufferers and their families the information they need to make their own choices about the most suitable treatments.

Other titles in the series

THE NATURAL WAY WITH

Irritable Bowel Syndrome

Nigel Howard

Series editor
Richard Thomas

Series medical consultants
Dr Peter Albright MD & Dr David Peters MD

Approved by the
AMERICAN HOLISTIC MEDICAL ASSOCIATION
& BRITISH HOLISTIC MEDICAL ASSOCIATION

ELEMENT
Shaftesbury, Dorset ● Rockport, Massachusetts
Brisbane, Queensland

© Element Books 1995

First published in Great Britain in 1995 by
Element Books Limited
Shaftesbury, Dorset

Published in the USA in 1995 by
Element, Inc.
42 Broadway, Rockport, MA 01966

Published in Australia in 1995 by
Element Books Limited
for Jacaranda Wiley Limited
33 Park Road, Milton, Brisbane, 4064

Cover design by Max Fairbrother
Designed and typeset by Linda Reed and Joss Nizan
Printed and bound in Great Britain by
BPC Paperbacks Limited

British Library Cataloguing in Publication
data available

Library of Congress Cataloging in Publication
data available

ISBN 1-85230-583-5

Contents

List of Illustrations

Dedication

To my parents

Acknowledgements

Heartfelt thanks to the following people for their help: Dr Peter Whorwell of the University Hospital of South Manchester; Andrew Vickers of the Research Council for Complementary Medicine; Roger Dyson, homoeopath and herbalist of Sydenham, south London; Stephen Church, medical herbalist of Coulsdon, Surrey; Simon Horner of the British College of Naturopathy and Osteopathy; and John Parkinson, acupuncturist of Putney, London.

Introduction

Irritable bowel syndrome, or IBS for short, affects millions of people worldwide. Some suffer mild symptoms every now and again, often during stressful periods in their lives, but others endure years of pain, misery and social embarrassment. In severe cases IBS can cost someone not just their health but their job and social life as well.

Yet despite its toll of misery, IBS is not a high-profile illness. Even sufferers are reluctant to talk about it. Bowel movements are an essential bodily function, like eating and breathing, and yet they are not a fit topic for discussion, even as we approach the end of the twentieth century.

This Cinderella image of IBS has, to a large extent, been promoted by the medical establishment. To them IBS belongs to a large group of baffling and time-consuming conditions known as 'functional disorders'. This simply means that something, in this case the bowel, is not working properly for no apparent reason. As there is no mechanical problem it must be 'all in the mind'.

That phrase has probably caused sufferers almost as much anguish as the symptoms of IBS itself. The sad thing is that it is not true. If you have IBS you have a real medical condition, the causes of which are only now just beginning to be understood.

Progress in the scientific understanding of IBS has taken decades of work by a small dedicated band of doctors who have to fit research around their already extremely busy practices. But progress is being made and a variety of possible causes has already been identified – few of them 'all in the mind'. What is becoming clear is that in IBS, as in all health matters, the effects of the mind on the body and the body on the mind are interlinked and we ignore this relationship at our peril.

Research indicates that, in order to 'cure' or even understand conditions such as IBS, conventional medicine must make the mind-shift towards the more 'holistic' approach of treating the whole to cure the parts rather than vice versa. Certainly the evidence is that the softer, gentler approach of natural therapies is more effective in IBS than anything conventional medicine has to offer.

This book aims to guide you through these natural therapies and to show you how you can start helping yourself get better.

Nigel Howard

CHAPTER 1

What is irritable bowel syndrome?

How and why it develops and who it affects

Irritable bowel syndrome, or IBS for short, is a disorder of the digestive system which affects millions of people throughout the world. Up to half of all people referred by their doctor to specialist clinics are suffering from IBS, and studies in countries as diverse as Britain, the USA, France, New Zealand and China show that as many as one in five adults suffer from the condition.

The severity of IBS is just as wide-ranging. At best it can mean a rush to the loo first thing in the morning and the occasional bout of constipation and tummy pain. At worst, the pain and upset of IBS can ruin people's lives, making them incontinent, shattering their confidence, and leaving them unable to work and virtually housebound.

IBS is not a disease in the strict sense of the word. It is a condition. 'Syndrome' is simply the medical word for a collection of symptoms that tend to occur together. In IBS symptoms such as stomach pain, constipation, diarrhoea and bloating are all the result of the bowel – the long, muscular tube that joins our mouth to our backside – not working correctly.

Normally the bowel smoothly digests the food we eat, gradually breaking it down into the vital nutrients we need and eventually passing the left-over waste out in the form of faeces, known medically as *stools*.

But in IBS something goes wrong with this complex and normally well-ordered system. As the name implies, the bowel becomes irritated. As always in life, irritation, if not soothed, leads to anger. In the bowel this manifests itself as tension, which results in the colicky, cramp-like pain felt by sufferers. These painful spasms gave rise to another name for IBS, *spastic colon*. Spastic is derived from spasm. You might still hear this name used, although its popularity is waning.

Anger, as everyone knows, is confusing. In the irritable and angry bowel, nature's complex and delicate system of digestion breaks down, and the result is the constipation, diarrhoea and the other symptoms so familiar to those with IBS (see figure 1).

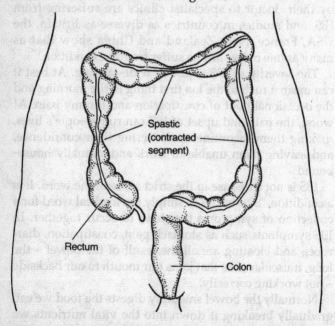

Fig. 1 The 'irritable' bowel

The symptoms of IBS

All sufferers will have some of the following:

Main symptoms

- Recurrent colicky stomach pain, often low down on the left, which is often relieved by passing wind or stools.
- A bloated, windy feeling, sometimes with accompanying rumbling noises.
- Diarrhoea, especially first thing in the morning.
- Constipation.
- Alternating bouts of diarrhoea and constipation.
- Small, hard, pellet-like stools which may be covered in mucus (and it is quite common to pass just mucus).

Other (secondary) symptoms

- A feeling of incomplete emptying after going to the toilet.
- Incontinence.
- Nausea, belching and, occasionally, vomiting.
- Back pain.
- Lethargy.

Of course, many people suffer from just one or two symptoms of IBS while an unlucky few have to endure most or all of them. Interestingly, many IBS sufferers say that the so-called secondary symptoms of the condition can be the most troublesome and life-disrupting, especially the lethargy and nausea.

These secondary symptoms can also complicate IBS in the minds of doctors who, as a profession, have traditionally been trained to compartmentalize 'illness' – which is what we feel – and 'disease' – the name doctors give to the condition that makes us feel this way. The results of this for sufferers can be unexpected and deeply disturbing.

Suppose, for example, you suffer from IBS with severe backache. It is the backache, not the upset in toilet habits (which you have probably experienced on and off for years), that sends you to your family doctor. Confronted with a patient whose prominent symptom is bad back pain, the doctor might refer you to an orthopaedic surgeon.

Gynaecology – the branch of medicine specializing in women's conditions – is also a very difficult area in this respect, as gynaecological problems are relatively common in those suffering from IBS. So the IBS sufferer goes to her doctor with stomach pain and abnormal periods and is referred to a gynaecologist.

If she is aged over 40 the chances are high that a *hysterectomy* – the surgical removal of the womb – may be considered. It is estimated that many women attending gynaecology clinics with pelvic pain have IBS and a proportion of these will eventually, after many tests, have a hysterectomy. In most cases this does not solve the problem and physicians treating IBS have a number of women patients who have had pelvic 'clearances'.

None of this can be classified as medical malpractice – everyone is doing their job thoroughly and obeying the time-honoured motto of 'better safe than sorry'. The trouble is that, although they are safe, it is often the IBS sufferer who is sorry!

The answer, many specialists believe, is better education and increased awareness among family doctors of the possible ramifications of IBS, so that, unless the symptoms point to a possible life-threatening condition, simple measures can be tried before the patient is whisked off for specialist examination.

What IBS is not

At this stage it is probably worth making a few points about what IBS is not.

While, in some cases, it can be potentially life-ruining, it is not life-threatening. The diagnosis of IBS, which should be made by a doctor to exclude the possibility of other problems, means there is no underlying disease, such as *cancer*, *Crohn's disease* or *ulcerative colitis*.

IBS is not an infection, although in some cases it can be triggered by a virus or bacteria. IBS is not a bowel inflammation like ulcerative colitis and Crohn's disease. It is not progressive. It is what is known as a 'chronic relapsing condition'. It is there in the background, occasionally flaring up and then subsiding, but it will not generally go on getting steadily worse.

Who gets IBS?

The answer is all sorts of people. IBS does not respect age, sex, social class, creed, profession or nationality. That being said, however, IBS does seem commonly to start between the ages of 15 and 40. Statistics indicate that more women than men suffer from IBS, but this could well be misleading, as women tend to have a more responsible attitude to their health and seek medical help for problems, while many men suffer on, not necessarily in silence!

IBS is extremely common in the developed countries of the West. About a third of the population of Britain have occasional symptoms and about one in ten have symptoms severe enough to take them to the doctor and to require them to take time off work. This has led to IBS being labelled as one of the so-called 'diseases of civilization' that are thought to have developed because of increasing affluence, the consumption of more refined and junk food, and less manual work and exercise.

Certainly it is thought that IBS is less common in Africa, Asia and elsewhere in the developing world, where there is less refined food – and often less food generally – and life is physically harder. However, as most people with IBS never consult a doctor – and many in the so-called Third World do not have easy access to medical services – it is obviously hard to obtain reliable figures.

What is certain is that in Britain and throughout the Western world doctors are seeing more and more IBS sufferers each year. However, opinions differ about whether the incidence of the condition is actually increasing. Some experts argue that there has always been a lot of IBS about but that, in the past, people put up with their symptoms because there were a lot of much nastier things to worry about first.

As one specialist in the stomach and intestines (known in medical circles as a *gastroenterologist*) puts it: 'These things are always relative. A hundred years ago when infectious diseases such as diphtheria and TB were killing people all around you, you did not worry so much about your irritable bowel. Now the great infectious killers are more or less under control people have time to tackle their other health problems.'

CHAPTER 2

All about the bowel and digestive system

How they work and why they're important

The bowel is a long, muscular tube running all the way from the mouth to the anus. It is lined with a slippery mucous membrane which helps food move smoothly along and protects the walls of the bowel from wear and tear.

From top to bottom the bowel is divided into the oesophagus (throat), the stomach, the small intestine (made up of the *duodenum*, the *jejunum* and the *ileum*), the large intestine (which comprises the *colon* and the *sigmoid colon*) and the rectum. When everything is working properly together this adds up to a remarkably efficient food-processing and waste disposal system known collectively as 'the digestive system' (see figure 2).

How the digestive system works

The first step in this intricate system takes place almost without us being aware of it. The thought, sight or aroma of food triggers glands in the mouth to start producing lubricating saliva – hence the common expression 'mouth-watering'.

Then as we chew the food it mixes with this saliva, allowing it to be swallowed into the oesophagus. As this happens a reflex action closes a valve in top of the

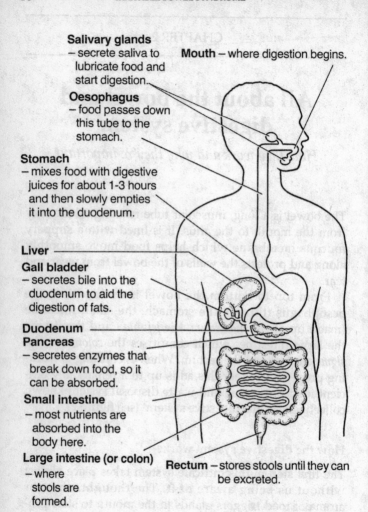

Salivary glands – secrete saliva to lubricate food and start digestion.

Mouth – where digestion begins.

Oesophagus – food passes down this tube to the stomach.

Stomach – mixes food with digestive juices for about 1-3 hours and then slowly empties it into the duodenum.

Liver

Gall bladder – secretes bile into the duodenum to aid the digestion of fats.

Duodenum

Pancreas – secretes enzymes that break down food, so it can be absorbed.

Small intestine – most nutrients are absorbed into the body here.

Large intestine (or colon) – where stools are formed.

Rectum – stores stools until they can be excreted.

Fig. 2 The digestive system

throat, called the *glottis*, to prevent food or drink 'going down the wrong way' – that is, getting into the windpipe and choking us.

The oesophagus is about 10 inches long and pushes the food down into the stomach with a series of powerful rhythmic movements. This makes it possible to eat and drink while standing on your head, should you feel the urge to do so!

In the stomach, acid gastric juice breaks down the food into its constituent parts of proteins, sugars, starches and fats. The resulting semi-liquid food then passes through a one-way valve, known as the *pylorus*, into the small intestine, which is more than 9 feet long. Here alkaline juices helped by bile from the bile duct, juices from the pancreas and colonies of friendly bacteria, which live in the lower part of the small intestine, continue the digestion process.

By the time our breakfast, lunch, dinner or whatever reaches the end of the small intestine, it has been reduced to just a few simple chemicals – proteins have been broken down into amino acids, fats into fatty acids and monoglycerides, and starches into simple sugars. These nutrients are then absorbed into the body through the walls of the intestine. Alcohol is the only substance that is absorbed into the body directly from the stomach.

The liquefied left-overs, material from our food which the body cannot use, passes on into and through the large intestine or colon. As it does so, the walls of the intestine absorb the water and by the time the waste matter reaches the rectum, ready to be expelled through the anus, it has become a solid but soft material.

Food is moved through the various sections of the digestive system by movements of muscles in the walls of the bowel. These contract and relax in slow waves in order to push food along, a process known as *peristalsis*.

The speed at which we digest food varies from person

to person, but generally the stomach is empty about two or three hours after a meal, and the small intestine after about four hours; the waste products are usually in the rectum ready for evacuation 24 hours after we have finished eating.

The digestion of food in the stomach and the small intestine also leads to the production of gas or wind, known medically as *flatus*. We get rid of this by expelling it either upwards if it comes from the stomach – by belching or burping – or downwards – 'farting' – if it comes from the intestines. Obviously some foods – beans are a notorious example – produce more gas than others during digestion, but the surprising fact is that nearly every healthy person produces between 3 and 4 litres of wind a day.

What can go wrong?

Obviously the digestive system is complex and, as with all complex systems, all the different bits have to be working in harmony if it is to function efficiently. Leaving aside, for the moment, problems caused by disease, there is plenty of scope for disharmony. If, for example, the walls of the bowel propel food too fast you get diarrhoea, too slowly and the result is constipation. If, for whatever reason, the muscles in the wall of the bowel contract too much too fast, then you suffer a spasm of pain.

The difference between a 'functional' bowel disorder and an 'organic' bowel disorder

IBS is what doctors call a 'functional' bowel disorder. This simply means that the bowel is not diseased in any way and looks perfectly normal but, for some reason, it functions abnormally. 'Organic' bowel disorders occur when the bowel becomes diseased or abnormal in an obvious way, for example when an ulcer develops.

What medical tests are needed?

When you go to your doctor with IBS he or she will probably arrange for you to have a few tests to exclude other disorders that can have similar symptoms. These tests may include:

- a blood test to check for *anaemia*. This is a reduction in the number of red, oxygen-carrying cells in the bloodstream which, despite popular belief, is only rarely caused by a lack of iron;
- a blood test to exclude *malabsorption*, a condition in which the bowel fails to digest and absorb foodstuffs, causing diarrhoea and malnutrition;
- a stool examination to check for internal bleeding;
- a *colonoscopy* in which a thin, flexible viewing tube is passed through the anus to inspect the bowel (figure 3);
- a barium x-ray. For this the mineral barium sulphate is mixed with water to form a white liquid that shows up on an x-ray, allowing the doctor to spot any physical abnormalities. It is either swallowed – when it is known as a 'barium meal' – to outline the stomach, or put into the anus – and called a 'barium enema' – to help in inspection of the lower part of the bowel, or colon. In either case the process is unpleasant but harmless.

Increasingly, however, as more is discovered about IBS many doctors are beginning to believe that these investigations should be kept to a minimum for everyone's sake.

After all, such tests are often uncomfortable and demoralizing for the IBS sufferer, who is generally much more interested in finding out what the problem is, not what it is not. Tests are also time-consuming and expensive. They are designed to discover the abnormalities found in other bowel disorders. But since in IBS the bowel looks quite normal, repeatedly sticking a telescopic viewing tube into someone's anus is unlikely to reveal the cause of it.

British gastroenterologist Dr Peter Whorwell of the University Hospital of South Manchester, a leading researcher into IBS, questioned a group of 20 long-term sufferers and discovered that, between them, they had consulted about 500 different doctors and undergone 128 major investigations and 53 surgical operations – all to no avail.

He points out that this endless round of intervention causes demoralization, anger and eventually despair to sufferers and also wastes a huge amount of money. He estimates that each person suffering from IBS for more than five years probably costs the British health service more than £4000 in tests alone – and that's without the cost of doctors' time at around £70 an hour.

A similar situation exists in every Western country. Add to this the cost in lost productivity through time taken off work and the cost of state benefit payments, and IBS is causing most countries in the West a vast amount of money.

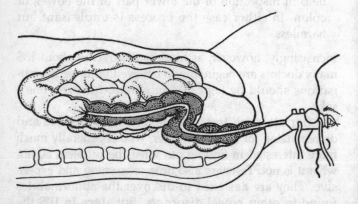

Fig. 3 A colonoscopy

Today, with people under the age of 40 who have no family history of cancer or bowel disease, many doctors will now diagnose and treat IBS without investigation. Older patients, however, may still need a couple of tests to exclude other conditions.

The 'Manning criteria' for diagnosing IBS

Doctors diagnose IBS if you have three or more of the following symptoms and other medical tests are normal. Remember, it is vital that your doctor makes the diagnosis of IBS so that other disorders with similar symptoms are not missed. Never try to diagnose yourself.

- Pain relieved after going to the toilet
- More frequent stools after onset of pain
- Looser stools after onset of pain
- Abdominal distension
- Passage of mucus
- Feeling of incomplete evacuation

CHAPTER 3

Causes and risk factors

How and why IBS develops

The straight answer is that there is no single, definite cause of IBS. The question has puzzled doctors and other experts for hundreds of years. Writing in the London *Medical Gazette* as long ago as 1849, a Dr W. Cumming expressed his bewilderment thus: 'The bowels are at one time constipated, at another lax, in the same person . . . How the disease has two such different symptoms I do not profess to explain.'

One of the biggest problems facing those researching IBS is lack of money, and this may go a long way towards explaining why the symptoms that puzzled the good doctor Cumming still baffle his counterparts nearly 150 years later.

Let's face it: IBS is not a 'sexy' subject, especially if you have not got it. Mention causes such as research into heart disease or childhood leukaemia and the money starts pouring in before you can say, 'test-tube'. When did you last see anyone in the street with a collecting tin for IBS research?

Things, therefore, have moved slowly, especially as it has taken the enlightened few many years to convince the majority of doctors – and there is still a long way to go – that IBS is a genuine medical condition at all. But considerable progress has nevertheless been made, and it now seems likely that IBS has a variety of possible causes, depending on the individual concerned.

All in the mind?

Orthodox medicine makes a distinction between physical and psychological causes of illness. But as research continues to add to our knowledge of human health this distinction looks increasingly unrealistic. It is now generally accepted by orthodox medical practitioners that a person's physical health has a powerful influence on his or her state of mind and vice versa. The two are so closely interlinked that it is patently nonsense to separate them.

Yet for years sufferers from conditions such as IBS have had to put up with doctors telling them: 'It's all in the mind.'

Mary, 54, is a fairly typical example. She has suffered with IBS off and on for nearly 20 years. She says: 'I keep going to my doctor but I begin to feel depressed as soon as I get near the surgery. I know the doctor will not want to see me. He looks depressed and almost starts writing a prescription before I have sat down.'

Consultant gastroenterologist Dr Peter Whorwell says 15 years' experience of treating the condition has made him 99.9 per cent sure that it is not all in the mind. But he says many doctors are to blame for convincing patients that it is all in their heads.

An IBS sufferer's first two or three consultations with their doctor are vital, he believes, often deciding whether a person will get better or will begin the endless dreary round of consultations, and examinations, so familiar to all too many. Whorwell says that taking the problem seriously is the first, most important step towards solving it. His clinic is full of desperate, angry people fed up with being pushed from pillar to post and fobbed off with the 'there is nothing wrong with you, Mrs Smith' approach.

He says: 'I let them talk for perhaps half an hour or even longer. These are very angry, hurt people. The important thing is that when they leave we have con-

vinced them that we believe them, that they really have
a proper, legitimate disorder. That is a good start. Once
they know there is really something wrong with them
they can start to cope with it.'

The 'all-in-the-mind' school of medical thought has
been sustained by two seemingly important factors. The
first is that IBS sufferers have nothing obviously wrong
with their bowel, such as an ulcer or cancer. In fact, IBS
is almost by definition a diagnosis of exclusion, the
'Well, Mr Philips, it must be IBS because we cannot find
anything physically wrong with you' approach. But just
because everything looks OK, it does not necessarily
mean it *is* OK.

Secondly, IBS is undoubtedly affected by stress. Many
IBS sufferers find the condition worsens at times of nervousness, anxiety and upset. But then this happens to
everyone to some degree, not just those with IBS. Most
of us suffer some stomach upset before exams, job inter-
views, getting married or other stressful events.
Anyway, some IBS sufferers actually find that their
symptoms improve at times of great stress, only to
return later on.

Researchers have long sought for links between IBS
and a person's psychological state. Some claim to have
found that IBS sufferers have higher rates of psychiatric
problems, such as personality disorders, anxiety and
depression. But other experts point out that these studies
involved people who had suffered from severe IBS for
many years and that therefore such psychiatric problems
could just as easily be the *result* of IBS rather than the
cause. After all, years of living with severe IBS is enough
to make anyone anxious and depressed!

Studies which look at IBS sufferers who do not consult a doctor about the problem – by far the majority –
clearly show that they are not psychologically different
from their healthy counterparts.

As a result, many experts now believe that IBS is an underlying condition, much like asthma, in many people. It is there in the background all the time, rumbling quietly away, and then something happens in a person's life which triggers an acute attack. Symptoms a person has ignored for years suddenly become important and this takes them to the doctor. For example, someone who has put up with the symptoms of IBS may suddenly become acutely aware of them when a relative is diagnosed as having cancer.

According to this theory, we all have some form of genetically controlled weakness which is handed down through the generations – and when stressful events happen the weakest part of the system is the first to feel the strain. For some people this may mean IBS, for others asthma, for others high blood pressure and so on.

Therefore, while a person's state of mind does not cause a condition such as IBS, it does influence how the condition is viewed by that person and what he or she does about it.

This does not mean, however, that occasionally IBS is not caused by a deep psychological disturbance, such as that resulting from physical or sexual abuse, in the same way that such a state of mind can cause all sorts of other physical symptoms. As one gastroenterologist puts it: 'It takes time and work on both sides but most of our patients get better in a year or so. They are not cured, they still get attacks, but they cope with them better. Some, of course, take much longer and with a few of these you might begin to suspect there may be skeletons in the cupboard – perhaps physical or sexual abuse problems – but you have to wait until they are ready to talk about it.'

There is also some evidence that people who consult their doctor about IBS are more prone to seek medical help for other problems as well, and this has led some researchers to put forward a theory of 'learned illness behaviour'. An interesting, if slightly bizarre, study undertaken in Cincinnati in the USA involved telephoning people at random to ask whether they suffered from either peptic ulcer or IBS and then questioning them about their lives and habits. This threw up some intriguing findings. Those with IBS reported more physical symptoms, treated colds and flu more seriously and went to the doctor more often for minor complaints than did non-sufferers. It also turned out that as children those with IBS were more likely to have been given presents and/or been allowed to stay home from school when they were ill.

The study's authors concluded that people who went to see their doctor about their IBS had learned while very young to associate illness with receiving attention and had carried this behaviour into adult life.

An alternative explanation, and one that fits in with Dr Whorwell's belief about the importance of having an identifiable medical condition in order to cope with it, could be that those people with peptic ulcers knew they had a peptic ulcer and had learned to live with it. Those with IBS, on the other hand, faced both an uncertain diagnosis and medical scepticism, making them more worried about their health in general.

Finally, there is the belief among some experts that IBS sufferers misinterpret ordinary bodily functions and conditions as somehow extraordinary. A classic example of the work that has given rise to this is a study by two US researchers, Lasser and Levitt, who, in 1975, found that IBS patients complaining of 'bloating' or 'gas' had no excess intestinal gas.

Others suggest that IBS sufferers misinterpret their bowel actions as well. They point out that a wide range of stool frequency, from three times a week to three times a day, is normal throughout the population. Some

IBS sufferers, they maintain, view these normal variations as abnormal and may also misinterpret frequent, lumpy or fragmented motions as diarrhoea.

Physical causes

So if IBS is not 'all in the mind', what are the physical causes? In this area nearly everyone has a theory.

Taking the conventional approach first, the vast majority of researchers believe IBS is the result of either a malfunction in the way the bowel moves food along – a process known as *motility* – or a problem with the way in which the nerves controlling bowel sensations work, or perhaps a combination of the two.

Food is moved through the digestive system by contractions of the muscular bowel walls. If the food is pushed through too fast you get diarrhoea, too slowly and you get constipation. If the walls contract too much the result is pain. Research has shown that the spasms of pain suffered in IBS are often associated with sudden clusters of contractions in the walls of the small intestine.

The results of other research suggest that IBS sufferers may have a defect in the way the nerves controlling the sensations they receive from their bowel work. People with IBS have been shown to experience pain at lower levels of 'rectal distension' – that is, when the rectum is less full – than other people do. Indeed, some experts put forward the fact that 56 per cent of people who suffer non-cardiac chest pain also have IBS as evidence that this defect may affect the whole digestive system.

The role of food

The bowel's whole purpose is to digest our food, and therefore it is only logical that what we eat must have some effect on its function.

Back in 1972 a study compared people in rural Africa, who ate a naturally high-fibre diet and rarely suffered 'Western' bowel disorders, with populations in Europe and the United States. It showed that the more fibre there is in the diet, the heavier the stools and the faster the whole digestion process.

Though, as most older people know, eating what was called 'roughage' has long been believed to be good for digestion, the results caused great excitement and gave birth to the famous 'fibre theory'. This holds that many diseases and disorders of the colon and other digestive organs, including IBS, are the result of a diet of refined and low-fibre foods.

Further research showed that fibre, in the form of bran, the husks of psyllium (ispaghula) – a member of the plantain family – or other bulking agents was effective in reducing constipation, along came the 'F-Plan Diet', and a culture was born. Soon everyone was shovelling down the fibre as fast as it would go.

Over the last 20 years it has become routine for doctors to advocate bran supplements as a first-line treatment for IBS. The problem is that while bran may be helpful in constipation, IBS is much more complicated and there is now a growing body of research showing that bran can make existing conditions worse. Even more worrying is the growing conviction amongst some experts that excessive consumption of bran – in the form of supplements, breakfast cereals and so forth – is actually creating more cases of IBS by aggravating existing, but mild, symptoms.

In a recent study of 100 IBS sufferers, 55 per cent said that bran made all their symptoms, but especially bowel disturbance, worse, while only 10 per cent found things improved.

Food intolerance

The role of food intolerance in IBS probably causes more heated debate than any other issue. Many doctors dismiss it out of hand while many unconventional practitioners base their whole treatment upon it.

Part of the reason for this may be confusion over the terms 'intolerance' and 'allergy'. If we find a certain food that does not agree with us we say we are 'allergic' to it, but often we are using the wrong term.

When our body's immune system discovers a foreign invader it sets out to destroy it. The mobilization of our internal defence forces and the resulting battle with the intruder can be monitored by studying the production of various chemicals in our blood. If the body acts as if certain foods are invaders and produces 'antibody' chemicals against them, this is a true 'allergy'.

But medical researchers have generally failed to find evidence of this sort of immunological reaction to various foods in IBS, and have therefore concluded that allergy does not play a role. Strictly speaking this is correct, given the definition of allergy, but there is now growing evidence that food intolerance rather than allergy may be to blame for many cases of IBS.

In cases of allergy only a very small amount of foreign substance is needed to provoke a quite drastic, even life-threatening immune response, as anyone who is truly allergic to foods such as shellfish knows only too well. But with food intolerance quite large amounts of the troublesome substance may be required and symptoms develop slowly and stealthily over days, weeks and sometimes even longer. Those who advocate food intolerance as a factor in IBS say many researchers miss this vital association because they fail to allow for this delayed reaction.

In Britain Dr John Hunter of Addenbrookes Hospital in Cambridge, a leading advocate of food intolerance as a cause of IBS, has suggested two ways in which this may work:

- First, as a direct effect of chemicals found in food, such as *caffeine*, *tyramine* and *histamine* (both found in cheese), *monosodium glutamate* and various additives such as *tartrazine*. All of us have to deal with these and other substances – many of them potentially toxic – every day, and to protect us we rely on chemicals known as *enzymes*, which are produced in our gut and liver. These promote the breakdown of such substances, rendering them harmless. But Dr Hunter believes that some people, perhaps for genetic reasons, produce fewer of some protective enzymes than other people, leaving them vulnerable to certain of these substances. Certainly research has already shown that many people with food-intolerance diarrhoea do not produce enough of the enzyme *lactase* (a condition known as *alactasia* or *lactose intolerance*).

- Second, as the result of an imbalance of the various bacteria, or *microflora*, in the gut. Dr Hunter's research and that of other laboratories shows that the balance of these bacteria may be extremely important. The microflora plays a vital role in helping to break down our food during the digestion process, but if some types of bacteria start multiplying rapidly at the expense of others problems can occur. Research shows that some IBS sufferers have abnormal balances of these bacteria, and Dr Hunter and his colleagues believe this may cause certain foods to be converted into toxic chemicals in the colon. These could then produce many of the symptoms of IBS, including bloating, intestinal gas, altered bowel habits and the painful spasms of the muscles of the bowel wall.

Antibiotics and other drugs

There is evidence that some people develop IBS after a course of antibiotics. Antibiotics are excellent at killing the micro-organisms which cause disease. The problem is that they also kill other, friendly, bacteria at the same time – so upsetting the balance of microflora in various parts of the body, including the colon.

These bacteria have a vital role to play not only in aiding digestion but also in protecting us against invaders such as the parasitic yeast *candida albicans*, better known as 'thrush'. The role of *candida albicans* in IBS is still disputed by many doctors, but some practitioners, both conventional and unconventional, have found that symptoms improve dramatically if it is eliminated. Other drugs, including anti-inflammatories such as *hydrocortisone* and *prednisone* and the contraceptive pill, can also have the effect of promoting the growth of candida and there is now some evidence that those stopping tranquillizers and sleeping pills after taking them for long periods can face similar problems.

Infections

Some IBS sufferers trace the onset of their symptoms to a bout of severe 'holiday tummy' or *gastroenteritis*, which is usually caused by bacterial infection. Again, upsets in the balance of the colon's own bacteria or microflora that were originally caused by the infection, and sometimes the treatment of the infection, may trigger IBS.

Hyperventilation and air-swallowing

Hyperventilation is fast, shallow breathing using only the top of the chest rather than the abdomen. It can occur at times of stress and tension and, in some people, can become a habit. It leads to breathlessness and, in some cases, chest pain, heart palpitations and even panic attacks. But hyperventilation also commonly causes gastrointestinal effects such as bloating and belching, because sufferers tend to swallow large amounts of air.

Are dental fillings to blame?

A small but growing band of researchers throughout the world believe that many of today's illnesses, including IBS, are caused by slow insidious poisoning from the mercury in dental fillings.

They argue that mercury can leak from dental amalgam fillings, and when it does it can interfere with the workings of the immune system and so kill friendly bacteria in the bowel, allowing overgrowth of candida and other yeasts.

Bio-Probe, a US monthly newsletter dedicated to warning of the claimed dangers of mercury fillings, pulled together the results of six studies in four countries involving a total of 1600 people who had had their amalgam fillings replaced.

Of those with gastrointestinal symptoms, 83 per cent reported general improvement or cure, as did 88 per cent of those who had specific problems with bloating. Generally there were reports of cure or improvement in 31 different conditions.

Before you book an appointment to have your fillings removed, however, bear in mind that, as yet, there is little hard scientific evidence to support this theory, and the treatment can also be very expensive.

CHAPTER 4

How to help yourself

Tips and guidelines for prevention and treatment

Suffering from IBS can be unpleasant, painful and very demoralizing, but this chapter aims to show how, starting today, you can begin to take action to heal yourself.

As with most long-term medical conditions, there is no magic cure, but thousands of people with severe IBS *do* get back to a completely normal life and there is no reason on earth why you should not be one of them.

The absolutely vital points to grasp right at the beginning are that if you suffer from IBS you have a proper, legitimate disorder – despite what some doctors would have you believe – which has proper, legitimate physical causes, and that, if you are prepared to accept this and are determined enough, there is a huge amount that you can do towards removing those causes and healing yourself naturally.

It may not feel so at the moment, but your body is a wonderfully balanced, intricate organism with a tremendous natural potential to heal itself if you will only let it. To take the first steps to unleashing this healing power all any of us have to do is to relearn something we instinctively knew as children, something so simple that we forgot it as soon as we grew up. We forgot how to listen to our bodies.

It may seem simplistic to say eat when you are hungry, drink when you are thirsty, exercise when you are restless, relax when you are tense, sleep when you are tired but, as adults, how many of us actually manage to satisfy even these basic needs? Instead, the increasing pressure of our everyday lives pushes along at a head-long gallop through disturbed nights and frustration-filled days.

All day long many of us sit hunched unhappily in offices in front of glowing VDU screens, far from day-light, swilling endless cups of caffeine-rich coffee and tea and snacking on chemical-rich and potentially toxic processed foods. After work our only exercise is walking to the car or the train and when we get home we spend the evening hunched in front of the television, swilling caffeine-rich coffee and tea and eating additive-rich processed foods. Then of course, to bed unexercised and full of caffeine and additives and, surprise surprise, we cannot sleep.

Add on the family and financial worries most of us have to endure daily, the tendency to perhaps smoke and drink too much, especially under stress, and, after a few years of all this, it would be amazing if we didn't get sick.

As we discussed earlier, we all have some form of in-built physical weakness, usually passed on from genera-tion to generation. The longer we go on ignoring what we really need for a healthy existence, the more likely it becomes that our misused bodies, like a car engine pumped full of the wrong type of petrol and oil, will begin to break down. And of course the cracks will start to appear at the weakest point. Welcome to high blood pressure or skin complaints and a host of other ills, including of course IBS!

Therefore the first sensible step on the road to recov-ery from IBS is a hard, honest look at lifestyle. Like any road, this road needs to be walked one step at a time, and if a general improvement in lifestyle doesn't work you can then dig deeper to discover more specific causes.

Diet

'You are what you eat' goes the age-old saying and, of course, it is true. (Actually, 'you are what you *absorb*' is even truer.) There is no doubt that a healthy diet helps you feel and look good just as an unhealthy diet has the opposite effect.

Foods that heal

The power of food to heal has been known for thousands of years. Hippocrates, the ancient Greek father of modern medicine – today's doctors still respect the Hippocratic Oath, even if they no longer take it – urged his students to make food their drugs, not drugs their food.

This principle also underlies traditional Indian medicine, called Ayurvedic medicine. This holds that some foods, such as meat and spices, create a more aggressive mental state, while others, such as dairy products and fatty foods, lead to a passive, depressed state, and yet others, such as rice, vegetables and beans, create a balanced, harmonious mental state. Ayurvedic doctors therefore prescribe various foods depending on their patient's symptoms.

The problem is that these days people are confused as to exactly what a healthy diet is. Huge amounts of publicity are now given to every new research-finding – it seems that what was 'good for you' yesterday is 'bad for you' today and vice versa – with the result that we are left reeling as revelation follows revelation, trying to find some sort of happy medium.

In this chaos, however, there are a few commonsense rules on which there is general agreement and which everyone, and especially those with IBS, should bear in mind:

● Whenever possible, avoid foods with added chemicals such as colouring or preservatives – which, in effect, means most processed foods. (Dealing with the chemicals that occur naturally in the foods of our varied modern diet keeps the bowel busy enough without loading in extra). Luckily this is getting easier as food labelling becomes more detailed. Remember always to read the small print on the label. Unfortunately, you cannot do this when eating out or buying from a takeaway. Takeaways pose a particular problem in this regard. They are best avoided, because often the cheapest, and therefore poorest quality, ingredients are used and, particularly in the case of Chinese and other oriental fast foods, potentially toxic flavour enhancers and preservatives, such as *monosodium glutamate*, are commonly included.

- Eat a balanced diet consisting of as much fresh produce as possible, low in animal fat, salt and sugar and rich in vegetables, whole grains such as brown rice, and fruit; this should be eaten in the form of small, regular meals.

- *How* you eat can be as important as *what* you eat, so always try to eat your meals slowly in a relaxed atmosphere and give yourself a chance to taste your food. Always stop eating when you feel full. Remember to listen to your body.

Fibre and IBS

The previous chapter touched on the increasing evidence that wheatbran may be counterproductive in IBS, aggravating rather than relieving symptoms for many sufferers.

However, an increase in fibre in the diet is generally considered to be beneficial for the working of the digestive system, especially in cases of IBS linked to constipation, as it lends bulk to the stool, giving the walls of the bowels something to push against (figure 4).

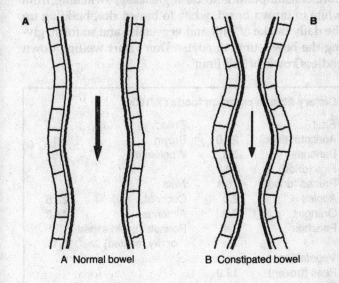

A Normal bowel   B Constipated bowel

Fig. 4 A normal and a constipated bowel

The answer, therefore, for those whose IBS symptoms do not improve, or get worse, with bran is to get this fibre from other foods such as oats, pulses such as beans and peas, and fruit. So if extra bran does nothing for you or makes things worse, don't panic and think that you might have a condition other than IBS. Try eating more of the foods listed in the box overleaf.

A spin-off benefit is that some of the fibre from oats and beans is, unlike wheatbran, soluble and there is a growing body of research indicating that soluble fibre can lower excessive cholesterol levels and so help protect against heart disease.

In any event, according to Simon Horner, lecturer in nutrition at the British College of Naturopathy and Osteopathy in London, the key to successfully increasing fibre consumption is to do it *gradually*, switching from white to brown bread, white to brown rice, building up the daily intake of fruit and vegetables and so forth, giving the bowel time to adjust. Don't start wolfing down endless bowls of 'All-Bran'.

Dietary fibre in common foods (%/100g)

Fruit		Bread	
Apricots (dried)	24.0	Brown	5.1
Bananas	3.4	Wholemeal	8.5
Figs (dried)	18.5		
Prunes (dried)	16.1	Nuts	
Apples	2.0	Coconut	23.5
Oranges	2.0	Almonds	14.3
Peaches	1.4	Peanuts (avoid salted	
		or dry roasted)	8.1
Vegetables			
Peas (frozen)	12.0		
Spinach	6.3		
Sweetcorn	5.7		
Carrots	3.1		
Baked beans	7.3		
Brussels sprouts	2.9		
Celery	2.2		
Potatoes (baked)	2.5		
(new, boiled)	2.0		
Cauliflower	1.8		
Cabbage	2.8		

Obviously *fresh* fruit and vegetables are better if it is possible to get them. Unfortunately most dried fruits are sprayed or dipped in preservatives to give them a moist appearance, and this coating needs to be removed by washing in hot water. Some dried fruits, such as apricots, peaches, pears and apples are often also treated with sulphur dioxide to help them keep their colour. Remove this by boiling the fruit in water for one minute and then discarding the water.

It is the same for changing to a healthier lifestyle in general. Gradually is the important word here too. Don't rush out to bulk-buy brown rice and lentils – it will probably put you off healthy eating for life! A healthier lifestyle means a healthier lifestyle for *you*, and it takes time to find out what suits you and your body and what doesn't.

Each of us is a unique individual and we each have different needs, likes and dislikes. A lifestyle that suits me would not necessarily suit you. However, many sufferers from IBS find that certain things tend to make their symptoms worse. The only way to discover whether this is also true for you is to try and gradually – that important word again – reduce your consumption of these things and see if your symptoms improve.

Remember that it is generally better slowly to cut down on things than suddenly to stop them altogether. Stopping altogether often just makes us want things all the more and, anyway, you may find that you don't need to banish a favourite food or drink completely.

Tea and coffee

Most of us are very fond of a cup of tea or coffee, but many IBS sufferers have found that cutting down, and sometimes even cutting out, tea or coffee or both helps reduce their symptoms. Try it yourself and see. You can try replacing them with herbal teas, unsweetened fruit juices – the sweetened ones are loaded with sugar – or spring water. Coffee and tea contain caffeine, which is a powerful stimulant. This has a direct effect on the functioning of the bowel and an indirect effect through general stimulation of the nervous system, which makes relaxation difficult.

Alcohol

As with so many things in life, there are pros and cons with alcohol. On the one hand, it is a depressant of the nervous system and too much of it can interfere with the proper functioning of the bowel. It can also encourage the growth of candida, which, as we have already seen, is believed by some practitioners to play a role in IBS. On the other hand, most medical experts agree that moderate amounts do not generally damage our health, and alcohol is an important relaxant and 'social lubricant' for many.

Again, the best thing is to cut down and see if it helps. Two good general rules, however, are:

● Never drink alcohol on an empty stomach.
● If possible, alternate your alcoholic drinks with glasses of water.

Our bodies, and especially our digestive systems, need lots of fluid to function properly, so making sure you drink plenty is a good idea – but, particularly for those with IBS, drinking large quantities of coffee, tea and alcohol may not be the best way to do it.

How regular drinking helps

American expert Dr Fereydoon Batmanghelidj reckons most of us are actually thirsty most of the time without realizing it. He recommends that we drink an 8oz glass of water *before* each meal – not with it – and another two hours after eating.

He points out that our bodies are 75 per cent water and only 25 per solid matter and if cells are starved of water they begin to function less efficiently.

Dr Batmanghelidj says six to eight glasses of water a day is the minimum we need to safeguard our health, and he maintains that good old tap water is just as good for us as the expensive bottled stuff.

Smoking

If you smoke, try to give it up or at least cut down. However little you smoke it is harmful, causing lung cancer, duodenal ulcer, bronchitis, emphysema and a host of skin problems.

Nicotine has a powerful effect on the nervous system and many IBS sufferers find that giving up helps reduce their symptoms.

Some people find it much easier to stop smoking than others but giving up is worth it in the end. Giving up makes you feel healthier, look healthier – if you are a smoker compare the condition of your skin with a non-smoking friend – smell nicer, a bit richer, and the sense of control it brings is an immeasurable confidence boost.

Relaxation

Relaxation, along with the ability to enjoy silence, is one of the forgotten skills in today's hectic world. Many people's lives are so out of their control that they never relax properly at all.

Relaxation does not just mean doing nothing. However you choose to relax make it a positive choice, and set aside a time for it every day when you can be quiet and alone. Try to find a minimum of half an hour a day to completely call your own. Whatever you choose to do with this time – some meditation, yoga perhaps, going for a walk, simply sitting quietly or even taking a long warm bath – this is your time, the time you take to listen to your mind and your body.

This is the time when you don't think about your job, your bank account, the children, the dog, even your IBS. At first this is extremely hard, as we all know how the moment we stop being distracted by outside things worries tend to flood in. But do not give up. Gradually it gets easier and you will discover that, by letting go, you actually begin to feel more in control during this daily period and more tranquil and relaxed afterwards.

After a while this daily 'set-aside' time will become both a refuge and a storehouse of renewal and strength on which you can draw for both the energy and the serenity needed to establish control over the rest of your life. Specific relaxation techniques and how to find out more about them are covered in Chapter 8.

Handling stress

It is generally accepted that the symptoms of IBS can be made worse by stress, and a considerable amount of conventional scientific research has been done into the effectiveness of stress management and relaxation programmes. Generally, the results are encouraging, as the following examples show:

● Thirty-five IBS sufferers were selected at random to receive either a stress management programme or conventional therapy including antispasmodic drugs. The stress management programme involved six 40-minute sessions with a physiotherapist during which sufferers were helped to understand the nature of their symptoms and their relationship to stress, and were taught relaxation exercises. Two-thirds of those on the stress management programme found it helped to relieve their symptoms and that they suffered fewer acute attacks as a result. Few of those given conventional treatment found it of any benefit.

● In another piece of research the number of consultations with doctors was measured before and after patients were given a six-month course in relaxation techniques. The same was done for another group of IBS sufferers given a course of conventional treatment. They were the 'control' group. Consultations in the relaxation group fell from 74 before to 6 after the course, while the number of consultations in the other group was 53 before and 41 after therapy.

Eventually you will be able to 'build relaxation in' to everyday activities and therefore reduce the overall stress and tension in your life. Even chores such as washing up can be transformed into relaxation if you do them slowly, with care and attention. When you clean your teeth, have a shower, a bath, a wash, or go to the toilet, do it slowly, concentrate on what you are doing and take the opportunity to 'get to know' your body and how it works. Are your muscles relaxed, how is your breathing and so forth? Learn what it feels like to be 'here and now'.

Breathing

Breathing is so fundamental to life – if we stop breathing we die – that most of us never really think about it. Only those suffering from diseases of the airways, such as asthma, bronchitis and emphysema tend to be aware of their breathing from moment to moment. And yet breathing incorrectly is an important contributory factor to all sorts of ills, including IBS (as we saw in the previous chapter with hyperventilation, which can both cause and aggravate the symptoms of IBS).

When we breathe in we take oxygen from the atmosphere down into our lungs, and when we breathe out we expel carbon dioxide and other waste gases from our lungs into the atmosphere.

This action involves muscles that lie between the ribs, known as the *intercostal muscles*, the *diaphragm*, which is the dome-shaped muscle that separates the chest cavity from the abdomen, and various muscles at the top of the rib cage and neck as well as in the abdomen and back.

There are two ways of breathing, depending on our situation and state of mind at any given time. Normal natural breathing uses the diaphragm. When we breathe in, this contracts, pushing down the abdominal contents and creating a vacuum in the chest into which air is

sucked. The downward pressure of the diaphragm pushes the front of the abdomen out. When we breathe out
the diaphragm relaxes, forcing air out of the lungs and
reducing pressure on the contents of the abdomen,
allowing the front of it to flatten.

However, when we get excited, upset or 'stressed' in
some way our breathing naturally changes. Instead of
using the diaphragm we use our rib muscles to expand
the chest and suck in quick, shallow drafts of air. This is
a good 'emergency' technique, as it allows us to obtain
the maximum amount of oxygen in the shortest possible
time, giving our body the extra power needed to handle
any emergency.

Chest breathing is fine as long as we return to normal
healthy diaphragm breathing after the emergency has
passed. But many people get stuck in chest-breathing
mode, which keeps them in a state of heightened tension
and can lead to problems of hyperventilation which can
include dizziness, panic attacks, chest pains, migraine
and gastrointestinal symptoms.

Watch babies and young children. You will see their
tummies push out as they breathe naturally using their
diaphragms. If they get upset or frightened this instantly
changes to chest breathing. When they feel better they
instinctively revert to diaphragm breathing.

In short, breathing, like so much else covered in this
chapter, is something many people have to relearn. It is
something they instinctively knew as babies but forgot
when they grew up.

Exercise

It is amazing how inactive most of us are. We spend
hours sitting in front of computers and television sets,
we drive to the shops and also take the car or bus or
train to work. But our bodies need exercise in the same

Breathing exercises

The ability to control breathing has been fundamental to yoga and most forms of Eastern meditation for thousands of years. Try this simple daily exercise. You will need a quiet room where you can be alone for about 15 minutes.

Undo any tight clothing and take off your shoes. Lie quietly on a bed or on the floor. Lay your arms down by your sides with the palms of your hands upwards. Spread your feet about 12 inches apart and close your eyes.

Listen to the sounds around you. Start with the more obvious ones such as those from other rooms, the distant rumble of traffic and so on. Now focus on the ones immdiately around you. After a couple of minutes begin to concentrate on your breathing. Do not try to change it, just concentrate on how you are breathing. Are you breathing with your diaphragm or your chest? Do you pause between breathing in and breathing out? How fast are you breathing?

Now slowly place one hand on your chest and the other on your abdomen just below your rib cage. As you breathe out allow your abdomen to flatten. Try always to breathe through your nose rather than your mouth. As you breathe in allow your abdomen to swell upwards. You are breathing with your diaphragm and your chest should hardly move.

Give yourself a few minutes to get into a smooth, slow, easy rhythm. Do not try to breathe deeply. Breathing in and breathing out should follow each other smoothly and slowly without any gaps or pauses. As worries and distractions arise do not try to block them out. Calmly let them float into your mind and let them float out again before focusing once more on your breathing.

Gradually your breathing will become smooth, calm and regular as you relax more deeply. When you feel ready to end the exercise take a few deeper breaths, open your eyes, give yourself time to become fully alert to the outside world again and then roll onto one side before getting up.

way that they need food and drink. The old cliché 'use it or lose it' really is true when it comes to exercise.

Without adequate exercise our body metabolism slows down. We put on weight, muscles lose their strength, toxins take longer to be expelled from the body and we begin to suffer all sorts of symptoms as a result, from headaches to constipation and depression.

The problem, of course, is that the less fit we become the more of an effort it is to do anything about it, and the longer we leave it the worse it is.

Admittedly the symptoms of IBS are not going to encourage anyone immediately to don their leotard and pound their way through an aerobic class, but regular exercise will undoubtedly make you feel better, both in yourself and about yourself.

So the key for those who do not feel up to games of squash and sessions in the gym is gradually to build exercise into your everyday routine. Take a daily walk. Leave the car at home whenever possible. If possible walk or cycle to work and to social events. Take the stairs rather than the lift, elevator or escalator. Do a few simple stretch exercises in the kitchen while waiting for the kettle to boil (some yoga stretches are very pleasant to do in the bath) or some running on the spot. And when you watch television, don't just sit there for hours on end – rotate your ankles, wrists, head and neck at regular intervals.

Gradually you will get fitter, looser and more confident about your body, and may feel up to a spot of swimming a couple of times a week and eventually, perhaps, a class or two at the local fitness centre. But of course by that stage you will already have had the satisfaction of knowing that you are fitter than the majority of the population anyway.

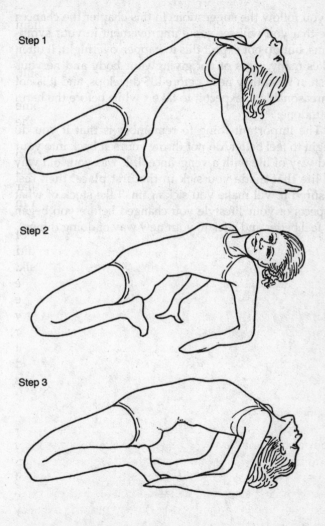

Step 1

Step 2

Step 3

Fig. 5 Yoga exercises useful for IBS

Give it time

If you follow the suggestions in this chapter the chances are that you will see some improvement in your symptoms, but do not expect this to happen overnight. It often takes many years of not giving your body and nervous system what they need before IBS develops, and it is not unreasonable to expect it to take a while before the harm is undone.

The important thing to remember is that if you do begin to feel better, do not throw yourself back into your old way of life with a vengeance. If it was your old way of life that made you sick in the first place, then rest assured it will make you sick again. Take stock of what aspects of your lifestyle you changed before you began to feel better and stick to your new way of doing things.

CHAPTER 5

Conventional medical treatments

What your doctor will probably say and do

Gastroenterologist Dr John Hunter, who specializes in the role of food intolerance in IBS (dealt with in detail in chapter 6), has stated that IBS is the most common problem faced by himself and other doctors, and it is also the one they treat most badly.

Certainly medical science has been baffled by IBS for centuries. Perhaps the main reason for this is the 'pigeon-holing' doctors have always adopted as a way of sorting out and making sense of the vast variety of human illness.

This narrow approach has benefits. For example, it provides a framework for teaching and for investigating illness and concentrates research efforts along potentially productive lines. It is doubtful whether many of the relatively recent strides in identifying disease-causing bacteria and other infectious agents and the development of drugs to combat them would have been achieved as quickly as they have without this approach.

However, with a condition such as IBS, which has a multitude of possible causes varying from individual to individual and which does not involve any obvious physical disease, the system comes unstuck.

Confronted by a patient who is hurting and angry and miserable for no apparent physical reason, our conventionally trained medical doctor is at a loss. With a packed waiting room, he or she seldom has time to listen to the patient's life story, or even a bit of it – which is a pity, because if he did he might get some idea about what is really causing all this pain and suffering!

An interesting piece of research from Sweden shows this only too clearly. IBS sufferers given eight sessions of simple supportive listening and advice about lifestyle had fewer symptoms and disability – both physical and psychological – three months after being seen than a similar group who received no such help.

Instead, the best most doctors can offer is reassurance that the condition is not life-threatening and prescriptions for a few things which hopefully will relieve some of the symptoms.

Fibre

This is the first-line treatment offered by most doctors. The trouble is that it is normally in the form of bran supplements and, as we saw earlier in this book, this often makes things worse.

Bran can be helpful in easing constipation. It leads to a bulkier stool which allows the bowel to push things through more quickly. But how it became a general 'cure-all' for IBS is hard to fathom, as there is only very minimal evidence that it does any good.

The reasoning behind the universal prescription of bran in IBS has always been that it might do some good and in any case will not do any harm. However, studies are now beginning to substantiate what many IBS sufferers have been saying for years, that bran makes their symptoms worse. What makes it so surprising that this problem is only now being recognized is that bran is of course wheatbran, and wheat is one of the foods that IBS sufferers are most frequently intolerant of.

In addition to this potential intolerance, wheatbran is pretty coarse and irritating stuff, and is actually the last thing most IBS sufferers, who often have some sensitivity of the lining of the bowel, should be swallowing.

In contrast to the often detrimental effects of natural wheatbran, manufactured fibre supplements made from plant extracts have actually been found to be beneficial for many people, and so it may be more sensible to give these a try instead. These are slower than wheatbran to show an effect and a little patience may be required at first.

Manufactured fibre supplements

Brand of fibre	Made from
● Fybogel ● Isogel ● Vi-Siblin ● Regulan ● Metamucil	Ispaghula – a member of the plantain family of plants
● Cellucon ● Cologel ● Celevac	Methylcellulose – powder made from cellulose, a substance extracted from plants
● Normacol	Sterculia – a species of tropical tree

Drugs

The first thing to make clear about drug treatments for IBS is that they will only relieve some of the symptoms – they will not get to the root of problem and they will not cure you.

The second thing to remember before you even contemplate popping any pills is that there is no such thing as a drug that just does good. All drugs and medicines have side-effects and sometimes these are worse than the symptoms they are designed to relieve.

There is no universally effective drug for IBS. Just as sufferers' symptoms vary, so the effectiveness of the different drugs varies from person to person – as of course does the severity of the side-effects.

Generally doctors are becoming increasingly reluctant to prescribe drugs for IBS unless all other approaches have failed. When they do prescribe what they prescribe depends on a sufferer's symptoms.

For example, if diarrhoea is the main problem, and perhaps incontinence is a serious handicap, then an antidiarrhoeal such as *loperamide* can be effective. Loperamide is an opiate which works by slowing down the working of the bowel, but it should only be taken in small doses for short periods of time, as it is an addictive drug and can also cause rashes.

For constipation that is not helped by increasing the amount of fibre in the diet there is a wide range of laxatives available, but again these should only be used for short periods of time. They have a tendency to make the muscles of the bowel lazy, so that when treatment stops the problem is worse than before.

Laxatives are divided into two main types:

- *Osmotic.* Osmotics ease constipation by drawing fluid into the bowel and so softening the stools. They should be taken with plenty of water and it is important to make sure you continue to drink a lot of fluid throughout a course of treatment.
- *Stimulant.* Stimulant laxatives work by increasing the constricting and relaxing motion of the muscles in the bowel wall, the action known as *motility*, in order to push the stools through faster. The problem is that this stimulation can aggravate and even trigger the pain often felt in IBS by causing spasm of the bowel muscles.

If painful spasms are the predominant symptom a doctor may prescribe a drug to help prevent spasms in the muscles of the bowel wall. These antispasmodics vary from preparations of peppermint oil (a powerful natural antispasmodic) to a range of complex and powerful drugs known as *anticholinergics*. The latter are effective, but their side-effects can include constipation, nausea, vomiting, impaired vision, a dry mouth, mental confusion and insomnia. Newer versions of these drugs are claimed to have fewer side-effects, however.

Some doctors also prescribe *anti-depressants* to IBS sufferers who have chronic pain, but it is far from clear just how effective this is. Even when anti-depressants seem to help pain, doctors are not sure why. Is it because of the drug's anti-depressant properties? Does the drug help prevent muscle spasms in the bowel wall? Or does it have a direct affect on how pain is perceived? At the moment, no one knows.

And, of course, as with the other drugs used in IBS, anti-depressants do not solve the underlying problem. What happens when a sufferer stops taking them and the symptoms return?

Some doctors prescribe short courses of tranquillizers, known as *anxiolytics* (such as *benzodiazepines*), when IBS symptoms are accompanied by anxiety and panic attacks. These may be useful if some particularly traumatic event has temporarily made someone's symptoms very much worse, but they are best avoided. These drugs can be addictive if used for any length of time, coming off them can cause a rebound effect of heightened anxiety and panic, and there is a risk that they may interact with other medicines you might be taking.

Obviously one of the chief problems of drug treatments in IBS is the very real risk of relieving one set of symptoms only to find that in doing so you have caused or aggravated another. On balance, then, unless you have a symptom that is particularly acute and troublesome, it is better to try and avoid drugs altogether.

CHAPTER 6

Food problems and special diets

The food alternative to drugs for IBS

In chapter 3 we looked at the reasons why intolerance of certain foods might well have an important role in IBS. Here the aim is to show how you can safely discover whether your symptoms may be food-related in this way.

This short chapter is placed between those on conventional and natural therapies because the food intolerance approach straddles both. It is a 'natural' therapy as it involves trying to alter the course of illness using food rather than drugs. On the other hand it is a conventional medical approach in that there is now a small, but growing, number of doctors practising in this way.

There is certainly an increasing body of evidence to show that tackling food intolerance gives long-term relief to many IBS sufferers. Cambridge specialist Dr John Hunter and colleagues checked up on 173 people with IBS whom they had finished treating between 2 and 39 months earlier. Of these, 165 said they were still benefiting from their new diet, while of those treated between 22 and 39 months previously 53 out of 61 were still well.

A warning on dieting

Gastroenterologist Dr John Hunter, a pioneer in the medical investigation of food intolerances, believes that it is only safe to tackle food intolerance in IBS under the supervision of a qualified specialist. He says a growing number of sufferers, dissatisfied with the general disbelief of the scientific establishment, are now consulting unqualified practitioners about the issue.

Dr Hunter warns that this can be unsafe if such practitioners use techniques like *cytotoxic tests*, *hair analysis* and *Vega machines* – all of which, he maintains, have been shown to be unreliable ways of discovering which foods are to blame. He claims that, as a result, a growing number of IBS sufferers now arrive at hospital outpatient departments sick and malnourished following diets which are nutritionally inadequate.

Exclusion or elimination diets

The only way to establish whether intolerance of certain foods is causing some or all of your symptoms is to follow a diet – normally for about two weeks – that excludes the most commonly troublesome substances, and then reintroduce the banned items, one by one, to see what your body's reaction is. This is known as an 'exclusion diet' or, sometimes, an 'elimination diet'.

The problem with such diets is that many of the foods IBS sufferers are commonly intolerant of are staples of our Western diet, such as cereals (including wheat, corn, oats and rye), dairy products (including milk and cheese), eggs, nuts, yeast and citrus fruits. So, if you are not extremely careful, cutting too many of these out of your diet can lead to nutritional deficiencies.

Of 182 sufferers treated by a team at Addenbrookes Hospital in Cambridge, 18 eventually had diets deficient in calcium and seven in iron. Three had diets deficient in vitamins A and D and two in vitamin C. One person's diet was eventually so restricted that it contained inadequate protein. A qualified dietician or nutritionist can find ways to compensate for this.

Also, if food intolerance testing is done properly it is a laborious business needing lots of self-discipline. Establishing a diet can take up to four months of testing, with the possibility of repeated unpleasant physical reactions as problem foods are gradually identified.

The message here is that if you are going to set off down the food intolerance road, fine. The evidence is that it can have lasting benefit for some people. But make sure you do it under qualified supervision and be prepared for a long, hard slog.

Study blames food

In one large scientific study of food intolerance 189 IBS sufferers were treated by dietary exclusion for three weeks. Ninety-one (48.2 per cent) found their symptoms improved and 73 of these were able to identify one or more foods of which they were intolerant. Some 14 months later 72 of these people were still well on a modified diet. There was a wide range of food intolerance although the most common culprits were dairy products and grains. The majority of sufferers identified between two and five problem foods.

CHAPTER 7

The natural therapies and IBS

Introducing the 'gentle alternatives'

For some people with IBS a simple change in diet and lifestyle may be all that is needed to banish their symptoms, but many others find they need a little extra help. So where to turn? By now you are probably all too familiar with conventional medicine's 'sticking-plaster-over-the-cracks' approach and are ready for something different.

Well, you are in good company. Each year in the Western world thousands of people turn to natural therapies for virtually every health complaint under the sun. The choice of practice and practitioner is in fact growing so fast that there is almost too much choice and, for some, this fact alone can prove daunting enough to put them off. Where on earth do you start?

Actually the first thing to realize is that if what you really want is the fresh approach of a natural therapy but the security of it being provided by a conventional doctor, that is by no means impossible these days.

More and more doctors are becoming converts to particular types of natural therapies and are incorporating them into their conventional practice. Dr Peter Fisher, a consultant at the Royal London Homoeopathic Hospital, who completed a study of complementary medicine throughout Europe in 1994, says that in the last twenty years what he terms 'the big five' – acupuncture, herbalism, homoeopathy, osteopathy and chiropractic – have become so common they are virtually orthodox.

This is even more the case in America and in Europe outside Britain. In France more than 80 per cent of herbal medicines are prescribed by doctors while in Belgium 84 per cent of homoeopathy and 74 per cent of acupuncture are carried out by family doctors.

But if your family doctor is not one of the enlightened, the next few chapters will hopefully provide an insight into just what is available, from whom, and what it can do for IBS.

What is natural therapy?

Natural therapy is based on the belief that the body has an inherent ability to heal itself and that the fundamental aim of any treatment is to bolster and enhance this ability.

Take this simple example. It is winter and you pick up the chest infection that is doing the rounds of the office, school or wherever. You go to your doctor and he prescribes a course of a drug, an antibiotic, to kill off the bacteria which are causing the infection.

A natural therapist would look at the problem from the opposite perspective, however, and would prescribe a treatment that boosts your body's defences, enabling it to fight off the invader by itself.

Back in the conventional surgery the doctor notes that the antibiotic has done the trick, the bacteria are dead, and your body is better. He has cured your physical problem and his job is done.

But, for the natural therapist, it is not that simple. He wonders why you were vulnerable to the bacteria in the first place. He wants to discuss your lifestyle, your general health and your state of mind. To him the whole person, rather than just the physical body, is important.

A surprising number of leading scientists have also recognized the value of this approach. Even Louis Pasteur, the father of modern bacteriology, on his deathbed uttered the immortal words: 'The bacterium is nothing, the terrain is everything.'

The natural therapist, therefore, wants to prescribe a course of medicine or action which will strengthen you to help prevent you getting sick again. For natural therapists believe that the human body is not simply a machine. Instead, it is a complex blend of body, mind and emotions, or soul if you prefer, any one or all of which can cause or contribute to health problems.

This 'holistic' approach was beautifully summed up by the ancient Greek philospher Plato when he said: 'The cure of the part should not be attempted without treatment of the whole. No attempt should be made to cure the body without the soul, and if the head and body are to be healthy you must begin by curing the mind, for this is the great error of our day in the treatment of the human body that physicians first separate the soul from the body.'

His warning echoes down the centuries and it is ironic that, some 2500 years later and despite all the advances of modern medicine, Plato's accusation is again being levelled at today's doctors.

It was William Blake, the famous English poet, painter, engraver and mystic whose work spanned the latter part of the eighteenth and the first part of the nineteenth century, who penned perhaps the best-known description of the fundamental principle of holism in his *Auguries of Innocence*:

> To see a world in a grain of sand
> And a heaven in a wild flower,
> Hold infinity in the palm of your hand
> And eternity in an hour.

Blake's view, like that of many modern natural therapists, was that the whole is greater than the sum of its parts and that the part contains the whole.

There are also a number of other important principles that underlie natural therapies and these are summarized as follows:

- True healing can only take place after the root cause of the problem is identified.
- Good health is a state of physical, mental, emotional and spiritual balance. This balance finds expression in Chinese medicine, for example, as the principles of 'yin' and 'yang'.
- There is a powerful natural healing force in the universe – the Chinese call it *qi* or *chi*, the Japanese *ki*, and Indians *prana*. Anyone can make use of this force and it is the natural therapist's role to activate it or help patients activate it in themselves.
- People heal more quickly if they take responsibility for their own health and play an active role in the therapeutic process – unlike the traditionally 'passive' role taken by patients in conventional medicine.
- Environmental and social factors have an extremely powerful influence on people's health and can be as important as their physical or psychological make-up.
- Each person is an individual and therefore no two people can be treated in exactly the same way.

Well, you might say, quite a lot of this sounds extremely sensible. Why don't more conventional doctors subscribe to these principles?

There are many good conventional doctors who do build up much the same sort of healing relationship with their patients as natural therapists and these physicians would subscribe to many of the above principles. But for the majority many natural therapies remain controversial because they are based on ideas that do not fit into conventional scientific understanding.

Reflexology, for example, involves massaging areas of the feet in order to stimulate healing in specific organs elsewhere in the body. Thousands of satisfied customers testify that it helps them but just try explaining why to an anatomist! The fact that a therapy appears to be able to defy the laws of science as they are presently understood, and still work is something many conventionally trained scientists are unable to accept.

What are the advantages of natural therapies?

Arguably the greatest of these is the relationship established between therapist and patient. The simple act of consultation with a good practitioner can be healing in itself. As mentioned earlier, some conventional doctors manage this with their patients but, unfortunately, they are still a rare breed. This relationship is often the key to discovering the underlying problems that are at the root of ill-health.

Another advantage is that alternative therapies, unlike drugs and most conventional medical techniques, are generally non-invasive and free of side-effects. This becomes an important consideration if you suffer from one of the host of conditions that tend to be long-term or chronic, such as IBS.

Conventional medical drugs can be effective at relieving symptoms initially, but there can of course be side-effects and sometimes problems of addiction. Also, with a few medicines your body may learn to 'tolerate' the drug if you take it for a long time, and if this happens higher and higher doses may be needed to gain the same effect, leading to problems of toxicity – in effect the amount of drug needed to be effective is enough to be poisonous.

Most natural therapies are very pleasant – especially those involving touch and massage. Many people who have no specific health problems book regular sessions just for the sheer pleasure and feelings of well-being these therapies bring.

While conventional medical drugs may have side-effects that can generally be described as negative, natural therapies have side-effects which are positive. Many people who try a natural therapy for a specific physical problem find as a result that they are more relaxed and positive about life in general and that their self-image is much improved.

How natural therapies treat IBS

Although all natural therapies share the fundamental holistic principles outlined above, in practice they can be divided into two fairly distinct categories, *psychological therapies* and *physical therapies*. The former aim to treat your mental and emotional condition while the latter concentrate on your physical state.

For instance hypnotherapy and meditation are clearly aimed at your psychological state, while manipulative therapies such as osteopathy and chiropractic are hands-on physical treatments for your body.

Of course, there are huge areas of overlap. Improving your mental state will help improve your overall health as well, either through the direct effects of relaxation or because you become more positive and change aspects of your lifestyle and attitudes that may be adversely affecting your health.

By the same token, improving your physical health will have a similarly positive effect on your mental state and emotions for, as we have already seen, the two are inseparable.

Then there are therapies which set out to treat mind

and body at the same time. Techniques such as *yoga* and *t'ai chi* are excellent exercise for your whole body but they also have a strong psychological component.

This global approach makes natural therapies ideal for IBS as it is a condition with both psychological and physical causes. For example, a psychological therapy such as hypnosis or biofeedback can help sufferers understand their condition and perhaps view it in a more positive way. This can get to the root of the problem or simply reduce the symptoms and help sufferers deal more easily with those that remain.

Meanwhile, a physical approach, say using homoeopathy or acupuncture, can both alleviate symptoms and stimulate the bowel to heal itself and regain its normal functions.

Natural therapies for IBS

Psychological therapies
- Hypnosis
- Biofeedback
- Meditation
- Autogenics
- Creative visualization
- Counselling
- Art therapy

Physical therapies
- Homoeopathy
- Herbal medicine
- Traditional Chinese Medicine
- Acupuncture
- Reflexology
- Massage
- Aromatherapy
- Yoga
- T'ai chi
- Colonic irrigation

CHAPTER 8

Treating your mind
and emotions

Psychological therapies for IBS

In the previous chapter we saw how the mind and emotions, which for many people include the concept of spirit, are inseparable from the body and therefore what affects one will automatically affect the other.

It follows that, for some IBS sufferers, therapy to treat their mind and emotions will have a profound effect on their physical symptoms.

Whether such therapies actually 'cure' the physical problem – our subconscious influences the production of the body chemicals which control the nerves regulating our bowel muscles – or whether they alleviate the symptoms by enabling the sufferer to put them into perspective is the subject of much debate, but at the end of the day it probably does not really matter.

What does matter is that many long-term IBS sufferers find that these therapies soothe away their symptoms and leave them feeling confident and in control of their bodies and environment, often for the first time in their lives.

Hypnotherapy

If you expect a hypnotherapist to wear a bow-tie and heavy glasses and to use a gently swinging gold watch you are going to be disappointed. Most practitioners using hypnotherapy are perfectly ordinary-looking, many are conventionally trained doctors, and most wear wrist-watches. A lot of them also work from rather uninspiring offices and clinics.

Most importantly, however, hypnotherapy for IBS involves putting things into your subconscious rather than taking things out. This sort of therapy should not involve any form of 'regression'. The therapist's job here is to place confidence-building thoughts into your mind, not go rooting around for dark childhood secrets.

Finally, proper hypnotherapy will not make you do anything against your will. You will not 'fall under another's power'. People undergoing hypnotherapy are aware of everything that is going on around them and are able to 'wake up' simply by opening their eyes.

Sessions usually take between 45 minutes and an hour. The patient sits, often in a quite ordinary chair, with eyes closed while the therapist talks in a steady, gentle voice. Gradually this encourages the patient to relax and slip into a mood in which he or she is open to suggestion. The therapist can then begin to convince the patient that they are confident, capable and are becoming physically well.

Most courses of hypnotherapy involve about 12 weekly sessions, and patients are given a relaxation and confidence-boosting tape to listen to at home in between.

As with other natural therapies, hypnotherapists hesitate to use the word 'cure'. Their aim is to reduce the number of acute attacks endured by IBS sufferers and to help them cope with those that do occur.

Nevertheless, the results of hypnotherapy, which is the most thoroughly researched of all the natural therapies, can be spectacular. Many centres report a success rate of more than 80 per cent and many people who have been virtually housebound because of severe IBS have

Case study

Helen Waters, 29, an infant school teacher from Manchester, who has suffered from IBS with constipation since she was 12, tried hypnotherapy at an NHS clinic as a 'last resort' two years ago after she became so ill that she had to take time off work.

She says: 'I was pretty nervous at first. I was reassured that it was a hospital clinic – I am not sure if I would have gone if it had just been someone's house.

'They gave me a medical examination first of all and said, yes, I had got IBS. Then they told me it was not all in the mind, it was a medical condition that could be made worse by stress. That was the biggest relief ever. That was pure therapy by itself.

'During the hypnotherapy sessions I thought they would be pulling things out of my subconscious but they put things in instead. It taught me how to control my bowel and stop the spasms. It also showed me how to listen to my body and pick up the signals, however small they were, that my bowel was ready to go.'

Helen had 12 sessions and used a confidence-boosting tape at home.

She says: 'Hypnotherapy was the best thing that ever happened to me. I am very much cured now and have not even listened to the tape for eight months. The discomfort and panic has gone. I don't know whether I actually go any more than I did before but I don't think about it at all. Life is completely normal. 'I have just got a new job and I am in the process of moving house and even the stress of all this has not affected me at all.'

returned to work and a normal life as a result.

However, a word of warning: Hypnotherapy is the only therapy in this part of the book for which it is preferable to seek treatment from a doctor. This does not necessarily mean that non-medically qualified practitioners are incompetent. But outside the medical profession hypnotherapy is poorly regulated and levels of qualification and expertise vary hugely.

Research

A number of recent scientific studies have shown that hypnotherapy can be an effective treatment for IBS.

- 30 people with severe, long-term IBS were randomly selected to receive hypnotherapy, psychotherapy or nothing at all. The psychotherapy patients showed a small but significant improvement in abdominal pain, distension and general well-being but not in bowel habit. The hypnotherapy group showed a dramatic improvement in all features, including bowel habit. When they were checked three months later this improvement was still present.

- 33 long-term IBS sufferers were treated with four 40-minute sessions of hypnotherapy over seven weeks. 20 improved, 11 of whom lost almost all their symptoms. Three months later they were still well. Interestingly, this study also showed that hypnotherapy in groups of up to eight was as effective as individual therapy.

Biofeedback

At first biofeedback may not seem like a natural therapy at all because it involves sophisticated technology. But all this 'hi-tech' is just another way of teaching you how to listen to and, eventually, control your body – a consistent theme throughout this book.

When a person is linked to the biofeedback equipment it provides them with information about their bodily functions. For example, their heart rate or brain wave patterns can be monitored and displayed on a screen. By making a conscious effort to change the display in front of them, people learn to alter these things in their bodies and, after a while, this can be done without their being attached to the machine.

Many IBS sufferers find that biofeedback can gradually help them to regulate their bowels and reduce the number and severity of painful spasms.

Meditation

This is arguably the simplest of natural therapies. It does not necessarily require a highly qualified therapist, although beginners normally need some assistance, nor does it involve high technology. But it does involve mental concentration and persistence and, for the beginner at least, some concepts that are difficult to grasp.

Meditation is much more a form of self-help than the other natural therapies. You can learn meditation in a class with others, but it is essentially something you do for yourself by yourself at home, without a therapist or teacher.

Meditation, in many different forms, has been used to quieten the mind since the dawn of history. All the great religions have long traditions of meditation, but its benefits have been experienced by saints and atheists alike.

With practice meditation enables you to gain control over your mind and emotions, enabling you to 'turn down or switch off' the endless clamour of fears and worries which beset us all. This control leads to greater mental stability and feelings of peace instead of panic. Being able to control your consciousness in this way allows you to direct your energy in more productive ways. People who meditate regularly say they need less sleep, have more energy, suffer less anxiety and generally feel 'more alive'.

Researchers have found that these beneficial effects on mind and emotions are reflected throughout the body. People meditating show similar physiological changes to those that occur in people during deep relaxation. These include a reduction in heart rate and blood pressure, a slowing of the rate of breathing and increased blood circulation to body extremities such as toes and fingers. There are changes, too, in the electrical activity of the brain and a fall in the levels of stress hormones in the blood.

The bit that beginners find hard to grasp is that all this control is achieved by *not* trying, rather than trying. This is a difficult concept, especially for Western minds trained to believe that the way to master a skill is to try harder.

When people meditate they are not resting or asleep. They are awake and aware. The aim is to free the mind from conscious control, to allow it to become empty of effort and to operate in neutral, to just 'be' rather than be thinking about something. To gain benefit from meditation you have to learn how to 'let go' and allow the quieter, deeper, serene part of you to take over.

Meditation is normally practised with the spine in an upright position and often involves concentrating on either your breathing or a *mantra*, a special word or phrase that is repeated over and over.

As mentioned earlier, you can learn to meditate in a class or, if you prefer, at home, as there are many good tapes and books available for beginners. The British Holistic Medical Association publishes audiotapes for relaxation as part of its *Tapes for Health* series.

Autogenics

Some IBS sufferers say this type of meditation can be particularly effective. Autogenics was developed in Canada and combines meditation with auto-suggestion along the lines of the famous mantra: 'Every day, in every way, I am getting better and better.' It teaches 6 specific mental exercises to encourage relaxation and creativity. Unlike many forms of meditation, autogenics needs to be taught by a qualified therapist.

Creative visualization

This is another variation on mediation. In this therapy ideas are introduced into the meditation. These can be either general images, such as beautiful peaceful countryside, aimed at inducing a state of relaxation, or they can be specific ideas targeted at a particular health problem. An IBS sufferer whose principle symptom is constipation, for example, might be encouraged to visualize a dam holding back millions of gallons of water. In the imagined scenario the dam would begin to crack and then break, releasing the pent-up water.

Counselling and psychotherapy

We all know how much better the simple act of talking over problems with a wise and trusted friend can make us feel and, at the basic level, this is just what counselling is.

There are times, however, when many of us need a slightly more professional listener than even our wisest friend. After all, friends are sometimes too close and too concerned about not hurting our feelings, and a professional listener will have a greater range of experience of problems and their solutions.

Counselling can be as simple or as complex as you like. Some IBS sufferers find it provides valuable short-term emotional support at times of particular stress and anxiety when their symptoms are bad. Others choose to use counselling – in its more complex form, called *psychotherapy* – to go deeper and explore unconscious issues and feelings. (It is worth pointing out here that psychotherapy has nothing to do with psychiatry, which is an orthodox medical discipline and often uses drugs and surgery to treat mental problems.)

There are many different types of psychotherapy. Freud developed *psychoanalysis*, which has given birth to the popular media image of counselling as something that is carried out by people with Eastern European accents and bow-ties. But today there are many other schools of psychotherapy available.

These include, to mention but a few: *Gestalt therapy*, which aims to work through unacknowledged thoughts and feelings using role play; *Rogerian therapy*, which allows the client to direct proceedings; *transactional analysis*, which investigates a person's relationships with others; and even *laughter therapy*, which, rather unsurprisingly, has been shown to be an excellent way of getting rid of tension and aggressive thoughts.

At its more basic level, however, counselling is now a well-organized and widespread therapy, and many health centres, clinics and hospitals have professional counsellors on their staff. As such it is hardly unconventional any longer but, like other natural therapies, it is safe, gentle and effective.

The important point is that it is up to you to decide how deep you want counselling to go and what you hope to achieve from it. Remember, the aim of counselling is to show you how to become more independent through assuming more control over your life, not to provide a crutch on which you may become dependent.

For details of how to find a therapist you can trust, see chapter 10.

Art therapy

Some IBS sufferers have benefited from this therapy, which aims to convert emotions into colour, shape or form. You can use any medium you like. You can rid yourself of desperate thoughts by hurling paint violently against a large piece of paper or by twisting clay into all sort of shapes or you can promote feelings of calmness and tranquillity through quietly drawing and painting.

CHAPTER 9

Treating your body
Physical therapies for IBS

This chapter deals with therapies which aim to release or enhance your body's natural power to heal itself. The therapies described below are all claimed to have success in treating IBS.

Homoeopathy

This is perhaps the best known of the natural therapies, partly no doubt because of the British Royal Family's much publicized use of it.

Homoeopathy was developed Dr Samuel Hahnemann, an eighteenth century German physician. He noticed that a herbal remedy for malaria, cinchona tree bark, actually caused symptoms of the disease, such as fever and headache, in healthy people.

Hahnemann concluded that symptoms were the body's way of fighting illness and that medicines that produced the same symptoms as an illness could help recovery. It was later discovered that cinchona bark contained quinine, the first drug to be used against malaria.

After experimenting on himself, his family and his friends, using weaker and weaker dilutions of various remedies, he noticed that the more the remedy was diluted the more powerful it became. Hahnemann had in fact rediscovered the ancient principle of 'like cures like', which was first expressed by the Greek physician and father of medicine Hippocrates in the fifth century BC.

How homoeopathic remedies are made

Homoeopathic remedies are made from plant, mineral and animal substances. The substance is first soaked in alcohol to extract the live ingredients. The resulting solution, called the 'mother tincture', is progressively diluted many times over in measures of tens or hundreds.

After each dilution the solution is vigorously shaken – or 'succussed' – and this is said to 'potentiate' the mixture, increasing its therapeutic power by transferring energy to it. In this way homoeopathic remedies are held to become more powerful with each dilution.

The final solution has a very low concentration of the original substance but a very high energy level. The solution is then dropped onto and absorbed by small tablets made of a neutral substance – though sometimes it is given as drops and even injections.

Hahnemann developed his discovery into a new system of 'holistic' medicine as an alternative to the conventional medical practices of his day, which included blood-letting and purging. These, he thought, were too harsh, often weakening the patient more than the original disease.

Homoeopathy today is still governed by Hahnemann's basic principles. Homoeopaths believe that the body has a natural ability to heal itself and that homoeopathic remedies stimulate this process. Therefore they concentrate on treating the person rather than his or her disease. They prescribe according to the individual characteristics of their patients and, as a result, two people could have exactly the same health problem and yet a homoeopath might treat them very differently.

Case study 1

Peter, a 51-year-old company director from London, turned to homoeopathy after 8 years of conventional medical treatment for IBS.

He says: 'I was in a complete mess. I had pain, bloating, terrible constipation and piles and everything I ate gave me indigestion. I was really angry at myself, my bowel and my life.'

Two months later Peter had finished his course of homoeopathy and his life had changed beyond recognition: 'My bowel is fine, the constipation has gone and so has the indigestion. I am sleeping properly and have unbelievable amounts of energy.'

Case study 2

John, a 37-year-old accountant, started getting symptoms of IBS 3 years ago. His bowel movements became loose and watery, he suffered excess flatulence and lots of rumbling and gurgling and his symptoms were made much worse by stress. He tried conventional treatments but without much success and, eventually, on the recommendation of a friend, consulted a homoeopath.

John says: 'It was amazing. After several weeks I was about 90 per cent better. My bowel movements were almost normal again and I felt generally better than I had for years.'

He returned for a second consultation and within a few weeks he had recovered completely and remains well.

Prescribing depends upon which 'constitutional type' the patient is classed as, and a homoeopath will spend a considerable amount of time during the first consultation trying to assess this. To do this he or she must build up a complete physical, mental and emotional picture of the patient – their likes and dislikes, hopes and fears, general health, sleeping patterns and so forth.

A course of homoeopathic treatment will involve several consultations over several months, and it is not unusual for the remedies to be changed during this time. It may take a couple of goes to establish the right remedy for you.

One thing to be aware of is the so-called 'aggravated reaction', which is the worsening of symptoms that sometimes occurs when you start taking a homoeopathic remedy. This is normal and shows that the treatment is working.

Herbal medicine

This is the grand-daddy of all medicine, both conventional and natural. Throughout history societies have discovered and harnessed the healing power of plants. Herbalism is still the most widely practised form of medicine in the world today, with over 80 per cent of our planet's population relying on herbs for health.

Even many of our modern conventional drugs are based on traditional herbal remedies. A good example of this is *aspirin*, which was originally processed from the bark of the willow tree. Another is the heart drug *digitalis* which comes from foxgloves.

Over the centuries herbalists have developed some quite elaborate systems of diagnosis and treatment. Herbs are said to have specific qualities such as bitter, cool or stimulating and which ones are used depends on which of these qualities are lacking in the patient.

Therefore illnesses thought to result from too much heat are treated with cooling herbs and those believed to be the result of lethargy with stimulating ones.

Modern medical herbalists no longer subscribe fully to these ancient traditions and are trained to use herbs according to their chemical and therapeutic actions. However, that is about as conventional as medical herbalism gets. It is certainly not a case of one disease, one herb.

Plants are said to have a particular affinity for certain organs or systems of the body and are used to 'feed' and restore health to those parts which have become weakened. As the body is strengthened its power to fight off disease increases. When balance and harmony are restored, the herbalist maintains, health will be regained.

Like the homoeopath, the herbalist will take an extremely detailed history of the patient in order to draw up a picture of the whole person, and the treatment of two individuals with similar health problems will not necessarily be the same.

Herbalists say their medicines are safer and more gentle that conventional drugs as they are produced from part of the whole plant, its leaves, berries, roots and so on. To make modern drugs pharmaceutical companies identify the ingredient in the plant that is active against the disease, extract it and mass produce it.

This results in extremely powerful and effective drugs. However, these drugs can be so powerful that some are, in fact, toxic to the human body – which is why they have so many unpleasant side-effects.

Herbalists say that this active ingredient is just one of hundreds and perhaps thousands of plant constituents and that the other constituents act as a natural 'buffer' to its toxic effects. Herbal medicines, they maintain, may be less powerful than conventional drugs but, because they are made from the whole plant, they are much safer.

Again, aspirin is a good example of this principle. It is an effective pain-killing and anti-inflammatory drug but its use is often limited because it irritates the lining of the stomach and can cause bleeding. Willow bark, on the other hand, rarely causes this sort of problem and, in fact, herbalists sometimes use it to treat stomach problems.

The herb *Ephedra sinica* is the source of *ephedrine*, one of a family of substances known as *alkaloids*. It is used in conventional medicine to treat asthma and nasal congestion. But it has the side-effect of raising blood pressure. However, within the whole plant there are six other alkaloids, one of which prevents a rise in blood pressure.

In the long run this means that herbal medicines may be as effective as conventional drugs even though they are less powerful. This is because people are often forced to stop orthodox treatment because its side-effects become worse than the symptoms of their medical complaint. In this way herbal medicine may well have a lot to offer someone suffering from IBS.

Herbal remedies for IBS can be as simple or as complicated as you need. Herb teas, available in most health food shops, can be surprisingly effective. *Chamomile* helps you relax and is a gentle antispasmodic. *Peppermint* is an antispasmodic and also has anti-inflammatory properties, as does *fennel*. Herbalists often recommend combining tea bags of all three to make a single drink to help soothe painful spasms and expel excess wind.

If you consult a herbalist he might recommend these teas, but might also prescribe *valerian*, which is a relaxant and antispasmodic for the whole body. Herbalists do not normally recommend taking valerian regularly – instead they suggest saving it for emergencies when your levels of stress and distress may be especially high.

Many herbal medicines used in IBS originated from

the traditional remedies used by the North American Indians. For instance, *cramp bark* is used to soothe spasms and relieve cramps. It is like a valerian for the digestive system. It also has a slight astringency, which is said to be effective against inflammation in the lining of the bowel.

Golden seal (see figure 6) is another North American Indian remedy. This is an antispasmodic, but it is also believed to act as a 'tonic' to the mucous membrane that protects the bowel wall, helping to heal any areas of damage. It is also said to promote the secretion of bile, which aids digestion.

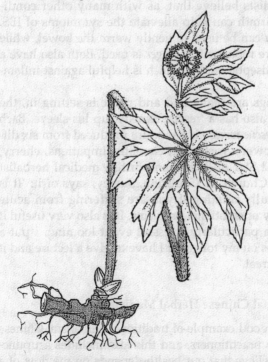

Fig. 6 The antispasmodic herb golden seal

Wild yam is also a North American remedy. It has strong anti-inflammatory properties and may be prescribed if you have a considerable number of painful spasms and are also passing mucus.

Liquorice is another powerful anti-inflammatory which also has laxative qualities. Herbalists use it in very small doses. Interestingly, liquorice was officially classed as a medicine in Britain until only about 150 years ago. Known as 'Pontefract Cake' after its main centre of production, its official mark of medicinal quality was its three castles stamp. The stamp is still used but has lost its original meaning.

Herbalists believe that, as with many other conditions, warmth can help alleviate the symptoms of IBS. *Cinnamon* can be used to gently warm the bowel, while for a more robust effect *ginger* is used. Both also have a slight antiseptic quality which is helpful against inflammation.

If things are really bad and panic is setting in, the herbalist also has a 'rescue remedy' up his sleeve. Bach Flower *rescue remedy* is a mixture produced from six different flowers: rock rose, clematis, impatiens, cherry, plum and Star of Bethlehem. British medical herbalist Stephen Church, of Coulsdon, Surrey, says of it: 'It is wonderfully calming if you are suffering from acute insecurity or emotional problems. It is also very useful if there is a particularly stressful event looming. I put a few drops on my tongue if I have to give a lecture and it works a treat.'

Traditional Chinese Herbal Medicine

This is a good example of traditional herbalism. Chinese medicine practitioners, and this also includes acupuncturists, believe that our health depends on the flow of a vital force or energy, called *qi* (pronounced 'chee'). This circulates between the organs along set channels, known as *meridians*. There are 12 meridians and each is said to correspond to the major functions or organs of the body.

Qi must flow in the correct strength and quality if we are to remain healthy. The Chinese herbalist will therefore use herbs to correct any imbalances in the flow of this energy.

In IBS Chinese herbalists believe that the spleen and liver must be balanced, the *qi* moved, cold cleared and blood nourished. To achieve this, cinnamon twigs with white peony root, astragalus and fresh ginger are said to be helpful.

Acupuncture

Acupuncture is the natural therapy for which conventional doctors seem to have the most regard. A growing number of them now practise it alongside their conventional medicine. However, most doctors practise a 'westernised' form of acupuncture which does not use the traditional Chinese medicine philosophy.

A large number of scientific studies have now shown acupuncture to be a good therapy for a number of conditions and to be especially effective at relieving chronic pain.

As we saw in the section on herbalism, traditional Chinese medicine has a radically different approach to our more familiar Western one. Instead of using herbs, the acupuncturist uses extremely fine needles – not much thicker than a human hair – to correct imbalances in the flow of *qi*. The needles are inserted at specific points along the meridians (see figure 7) and, depending on how the needle is manipulated – it may be gently twirled in place – the energy is either dispelled from or drawn to the meridian.

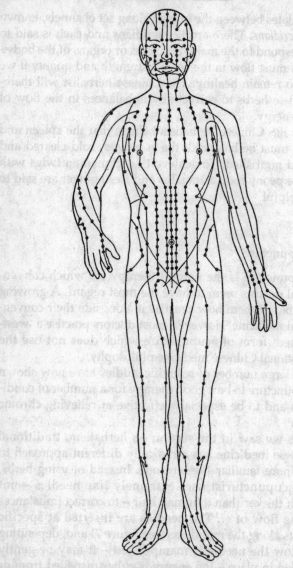

Fig. 7 Acupuncture meridians

Many people are put off by the thought of having needles poked into their skin. But the needles are so fine that they do not hurt in the way an injection does. It is quite possible to be completely unaware that the needles are being inserted at all. When a needle is inserted there is sometimes a feeling of heaviness. In fact, once they overcome their nervousness many people find the whole process positively relaxing and enjoyable.

Chinese medicine's system of diagnosis is also very different from the conventional Western one. The acupuncturist needs to assess the state of your energy and to do this will take an extremely detailed history of your general health. He or she will gain a lot of information about your health by examining your tongue, noting the colour and quality of your skin and making a special diagnosis of your pulse.

The practitioner will then decide whether you have a 'hot' or a 'cold' syndrome and whether this is caused by a deficiency or an excess.

Perhaps the cause is a deficiency of *yin* or *yang* – the balancing forces of the body – or of *qi*, or even of blood. On the other hand it could be the result of an invasion by a bacterium, a virus or a fungus, and this is known as an *excess*.

In traditional Chinese medicine there is no such label as IBS. A clutch of symptoms including abdominal pain, stools with blood and/or mucus, diarrhoea or watery stools, possible fever and thirst, a yellow sticky tongue and a 'rapid rolling' or soft rapid pulse might indicate that the problem was 'damp heat in the large intestine'.

On the other hand, fullness and distension, diarrhoea, sticky saliva, a sticky white tongue and a soft pulse could point to 'invasion of the spleen by cold damp'.

'Damp heat in the spleen and stomach' might be indicated by loose stools, intestinal fullness, stickiness in the mouth, a yellow sticky tongue and a rapid pulse.

The acupuncturist would stimulate points on the meridians to rebalance the energy and cure these problems.

Specific acupuncture points on the leg below the knee relate to the stomach. Stimulation of these is said to reinforce the blood and *qi* and disperse phlegm – a major cause of damp heat.

Points at the navel might also be used to increase spleen and stomach function, reduce abdominal pain and diarrhoea and generally improve the condition of the intestines.

Reflexology

This is a popular natural therapy and has a reputation for being helpful in IBS and in other bowel and bladder disorders.

Reflexologists believe that the feet are an anatomical map of the body. If you look at a foot from underneath it does seem to bear a resemblance to a human body, broad at the shoulders and narrowing down towards the waist and hips.

In reflexology specific areas of the feet represent certain organs and areas of the body. Therefore tension, damage or disease in an organ or body structure will be reflected in its corresponding area of the foot, known as its *reflex zone*. By careful massage of this reflex zone the practitioner can help relax the tension and so heal the damaged or diseased area.

Reflexologists examine your feet – the bone structure, the colour and texture of the skin, the tone of the muscles – to evaluate the overall state of your health. They can then investigate the health of individual organs in your body by using their fingers to gently press on the reflex zones. If the organ is healthy all you will feel is the

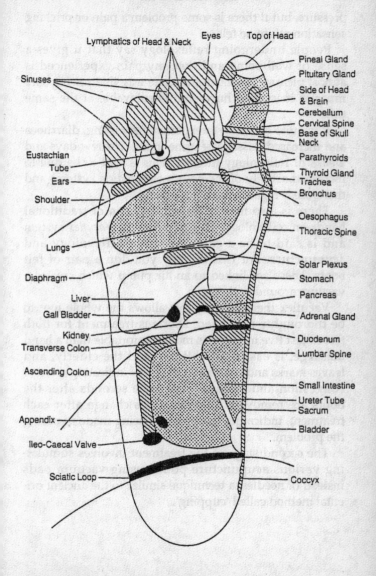

Fig. 8 Reflex zones on the feet

pressure, but if there is some problem a pain or pricking sensation might be felt.

People undergoing reflexology say that it gives a sense of well-being and that any pain experienced is almost pleasant, in much the same way that having sore muscles massaged hurts and is enjoyable at the same time.

It is quite common to experience sweating, diarrhoea and increased passage of urine in the first few days and weeks of reflexology therapy. This is said to be due to increased activity of the body's elimination systems and therefore is regarded as a good thing.

There is also now a 'hi-tech' version of traditional hands-on reflexology. This is called the *Vacuflex* system and is said to be a combination of reflexology and acupuncture. For this therapy you don a pair of felt boots. These are linked to an air pump which creates a vacuum around both feet.

Vacuflex therapists say this allows the whole foot to be thoroughly massaged, shortens treatment for both feet to just five minutes, is more comfortable than a hand massage, is easier for children and the elderly, and leaves marks and colours on the feet – indicating areas of congestion and disease – for some seconds after the boots are removed. These patterns change after each treatment, indicating the progress being made in curing the problem.

The second stage of the treatment involves stimulating various acupuncture points using vacuum pads instead of needles, a technique similar to the ancient oriental method called 'cupping'.

Case study

Ann, a mother of three young children, suffered from IBS for 15 years. Her attacks often lasted for up to three weeks at a time and caused intense pain. Antispasmodic drugs and painkillers from her family doctor had little effect.

She says: 'Eleven months ago, during the worst bout I have ever suffered, I decided to try a course of weekly Vacuflex treatments.

'That particular bout subsided long before it would usually have done and I have had no recurrence of the dreadful pain since. I have not needed to return to my doctor for any drug treatment for the problem and I have found that at times when I have recognized the warning signs a Vacuflex treatment has been enough to ward off an attack.

'I feel much less tense, my quality of sleep is much improved and an interesting spin-off effect is that streaming sinuses, which have plagued me every morning for as long as I can remember, have cleared up totally.'

Massage

Massage is another of the oldest and simplest forms of natural therapy and grew out of the principle that being touched in certain ways can be beneficial to health.

There are various forms, ranging from the basic physical massage, which aims to improve muscle tone, enhance blood circulation, ease stiff joints and work out knotted tissue, to so-called 'holistic massage', which sets out to treat the whole person physically, mentally and spiritually.

Holistic massage is gentler and more nurturing than

the more traditional forms. Its aim is to put you back in touch with your body, teach you how to listen to it and how to be happy with it.

Aromatherapy

Many people find this combination of massage and herbal medicine very appealing. Aromatherapists use oils distilled from plants, called *essential oils*, for therapeutic purposes.

Just as we all know what a powerful sense smell can be, recalling memories of past events and places, so certain smells can be relaxing and others invigorating. Smells can alter our moods, help us relax or perk us up.

But aromatherapists believe that essential oils have a deeper medicinal value as well. They maintain that some oils have anti-inflammatory properties, that some help reduce mucus, that others are good for the intestines and yet others for the blood.

In fact there is a growing body of scientific evidence that seems to support these claims, and certainly some oils have been shown to have anti-bacterial properties.

All aromatherapists are trained in massage and a massage with essential oils is the most popular form of aromatherapy. The massage is relaxing and healing for your body while the essential oils are absorbed into your body through the skin.

But aromatherapy uses essential oils in a variety of other ways too. Oils can be burned so that the vapour fills the room, added to a bowl of hot water near a radiator, and used in baths and inhalations.

Yoga

Yoga is an ancient Indian system of body and breathing exercises which aims to promote physical health and harmonize an individual's mind, body and emotions. It is designed to improve muscle tone, increase suppleness, massage the internal organs and promote better breathing and blood circulation.

The aim is also to improve the flow of vital life energy – the Indians call it *prana* – through the body, thus retaining balance and good health. People who regularly practise yoga exercises say they feel fitter, lighter, less anxious and more confident.

Scientific studies have confirmed the benefit of yoga in a wide range of conditions and there are specific exercises which can help improve bowel function.

But yoga is more than just a collection of daily exercises, however beneficial they may be. It is a philosophy and, to the dedicated, a way of life.

Both meditation and diet are of great importance. Yogis (yoga masters) believe that only foods that increase vitality, energy and clear thought should be eaten. Foods which lead to depression, lethargy or dependence – such as processed foods, coffee and alcohol – should be avoided, as should those which lead to stimulation – such as rich, spicy foods.

The aim of the yoga lifestyle is to live a calm and well-ordered life. Surroundings and clothes should be kept clean and as simple as possible and all types of excess, over-indulgence, violence and untruth avoided.

T'ai chi

Often described as martial arts without violence, t'ai chi originated in China thousands of years ago. It is based on the Taoist philosophy of 'yin' and 'yang', the two balancing forces in the universe. The Chinese believe that the best way to live a healthy, happy life is to interfere with this balance as little as possible.

In keeping with this philosophy, t'ai chi exercises are

designed to flow gently and naturally from one to the other, so that each movement is created by its predecessor and does not need any separate effort. This lack of effort means there is less disturbance to the natural balance of universal forces. Exercises follow a precise pattern, known as the *form*, and this has to be learned with a teacher.

Those who practice t'ai chi regularly – it can be done alone or in pairs – say it brings a sense of peace and well-being, teaches balance and poise, builds strength and improves the powers of concentration.

Colonic irrigation

Also known as colonic hydrotherapy, this is a sort of 'internal bath'. It involves inserting into the rectum a small hose-like device with two tubes – one which pumps water in and another which draws it out again.

Exponents say that the process cleanses the colon of poisons and accumulated faecal matter and so helps restore healthy bowel function. But it is not without dangers and risks, and practitioners need to be both skilled and knowledgeable. A high degree of hygiene is vital.

Opinions vary about whether colonic irrigation has any benefit in IBS. Certainly it has not been the subject of any specific trials for IBS so far.

CHAPTER 10

How to find and choose a natural therapist

Tips and guidelines for finding reliable help

It is unfortunately not as easy as it should be to find the right therapist. Although natural medicine is enjoying a boom and everyone seems to want to use it, diversity, competition between groups and duplication within therapies has made the task a difficult one in most countries in which natural medicine is growing in popularity.

It is the main purpose of *The Natural Way* series to help you find the right gentle therapy for your condition – but finding the right practitioner or therapist is in some ways the hardest task.

The best answer is almost always personal recommendation, and this applies as much to doctors as to non-medical practitioners. Go to someone a friend or somebody you trust has recommended. As a rule of thumb it cannot be bettered. But if you still cannot get a recommendation, what next? There are several options:

● Go to your local doctor's clinic or health centre and ask their advice. It may take some courage and you may not get a sympathetic response, but it is worth a try, and you may get a pleasant surprise: you may find they have the very person you need – either someone who works at the clinic or someone to whom patients are referred (which means, in countries with a state health service, possibly free treatment).

- Your nearest natural health centre may be able to help, or even a natural health practitioner who you know is not the right person for you but who may be prepared to recommend someone else. This is not as good as personal recommendation, but therapists who specialize in natural therapy tend to know who else is at work in their area and, more important, who is any good. You can get the names of centres and individual practitioners to approach from health food shops, local directories or local listings in newspapers, magazines, citizens' advice and information centres, and libraries. If you are into computers and have a modem, computer networks have lists. A particularly good bet is a natural health centre in your area which has several practitioners with different skills working at it. The better centres have a system where a patient contacting them for help will be offered a consultation in which his or her case is considered by a panel of practitioners, and a therapy (or therapies) and therapist (or therapists) are recommended. Such an approach is still in its infancy, though, so it may be hard to find.

- Failing a local recommendation or the availability of an enlightened group practice, the next step is to contact any of the national therapy 'umbrella' organizations and ask for their list(s) of registered organizations or practitioners. Their addresses are listed in Appendix A. They may charge for their lists (especially for postage and packing) and may also charge separately not only for individual therapies but also – because there is still no one recognized organization for each therapy in many countries – for individual organizations within therapies. If you can afford it ask for the lot.

---

10 ways of finding a therapist

- Word-of-mouth (usually the best method)
- Your local family medical centres
- Your local natural health centres
- Your local health food shops
- Health farms and beauty treatment centres
- Local patient support groups
- National therapy organizations (but see opposite)
- Computer networks (you need a modem)
- Public libraries and information centres
- Local directories, newspapers and magazines

Checking professional organizations

Whether or not you have found a therapist straight away it is still a good idea to check on his or her professional background. This becomes almost essential if you are picking a name from a list rather than following a recommendation from a friend. Just because a therapist belongs to an organization doesn't mean that he or she comes with a guarantee. Some organizations do no more vetting of their members than making sure they have paid their membership fees.

The first thing to do is to check the status of the individual associations or professional organizations whose names you have got. A good association will publish the information clearly and simply in the same booklet as its membership list. Few seem to, however, and so you may have to ring them up or write to them. The following are the sort of questions you should try and get answered:

- When was the association founded? (Groups spring up all the time and you may find it useful to know if they have been going 50 years or started yesterday.)
- How many members does it have? (Size will give you a good idea of its public acceptance and genuine aims.)

- Is it a charity or educational trust – with a formal constitution, an elected committee and published accounts – or is it a private limited company? (Private companies can be secretive and self-serving.)
- Is it part of a larger network of professional organizations? (Groups that go their own way are, on balance, more suspect than those who 'join in'.)
- Does the association have a code of ethics, complaints mechanism and disciplinary procedures? If so, what are they?
- Is the association linked to one particular school or college? (One that is may have no independent assessment of its membership; the head of the association may also be the head of the college.)
- What are the criteria for membership? (If it is graduation from one particular school or college, the same problem arises as above.)
- Are members covered by professional indemnity insurance against accident and malpractice?

Checking training and qualifications

Next you may want to try and satisfy yourself about their training and qualifications. A good listing will, again, describe the qualifications and say what the initials after every member's name mean. Yet again, few seem to. So it's a case of ringing or writing to find out. Questions to ask are the following:

- How long is the training?
- Is it full-time or part-time?
- Does it include seeing patients under supervision?
- Is the qualification recognised?
- If so, by whom?

The British Medical Association's opinion

In its long-awaited second report into the practice of natural medicine in Britain, published in June 1993, the British Medical Association recommended that anyone seeking the help of a non-conventional therapist – doctor or patient – should ask the following questions:

- Is the therapist registered with a professional organization?
- Does the professional organization have the following:
  - a public register?
  - a code of practice?
  - an effective disciplinary procedure and sanction?
  - a complaints mechanism?
- What qualification does the therapist hold?
- What training was involved in getting the qualification(s)?
- How many years has the therapist been practising?
- Is the therapist covered by professional indemnity insurance?

The BMA said that although it would like to see natural therapies regulated by law, with a single regulating body for each therapy, it did not think that all therapies needed regulating. For the majority, it said, 'the adoption of a code of practice, training structures and voluntary registration would be sufficient'.

Complementary Medicine: New Approaches to Good Practice (Oxford University Press, 1993)

Making the choice

The final choice is a matter of using a combination of common sense and intuition and giving someone a try. But do not hesitate to double-check with them when you see them that the information in the listing agrees with what they tell you – nor to cancel an appointment (give at least 24 hours' notice if you can) or to walk out if you do not like anything about the person, the place or the treatment. The important advice at all times is to ask questions, as many as you need to, and use your intuition. Never forget: it's your body and mind!

What it's like seeing a natural therapist

In a word, different. But it is also very natural. Since most therapists, even those in countries with state health systems, still work privately for the most part, there is no established uniform or common outlook. Though they may all share, more or less, a belief in the principles outlined in chapter 7, you are liable to come across individuals as different as chalk from cheese, representing all walks of life, from the rich to the poor, the politically left to the politically right. That means you will come across as much variety in dress, thinking and behaviour as there are fashions, from the elegant and formal to the positively informal and 'woolly-haired' (though, for image reasons, many now wear a white coat to look more like a doctor!).

Equally, you will find their premises very different – reflecting their attitudes to their work and the world. Some will present a 'brass plaque' image, working in a clinic or room away from home with receptionist and brisk efficiency, while others will see you in their living-room, surrounded by pot plants and domestic clutter. Remember, though, image may be some indication of status but it is little guarantee of ability. You are as likely to find a therapist of quality working from home as one in a formal clinic.

There are some characteristics, however – probably the most important ones – that you will find common to all natural therapists.

● They will give you far more time than you are used to with a family doctor. An initial consultation will rarely last less than an hour, and often longer. During it they will ask you all about yourself so they can form a proper understanding of what makes you tick and what may be the fundamental cause(s) of your problem.

- They will charge for their time and for any remedies they prescribe, which they may well sell from their own stocks. But many therapists offer reduced fees, and even waive fees altogether, for deserving causes or for people who genuinely cannot afford it.

Sensible precautions

- Though most practitioners practise for fees, no ethical person will ask for fees in advance of treatment unless for special tests or medicines, but even this is unusual. If you are asked for 'down-payments' of any sort ask exactly what they are for and if you don't like the reasons refuse to pay.
- Be sceptical of anyone who 'guarantees' you a cure. No one can (not even doctors).
- Be very wary of stopping drugs prescribed by your family doctor on the therapist's insistence without first talking things over with your doctor. Non-medical therapists know little about pharmaceutical drugs and there may be a danger to yourself if you stop suddenly or without preparation.
- If you are female feel free to have someone with you if you need to undress and if being accompanied makes you feel more comfortable. No ethical therapist will refuse such a request, and if they do have nothing more to do with them.

What to do if things go wrong

The most important thing to decide is whether you think the therapist has done his or her absolute best to get you better without hurting or harming you in any way. Failure to cure you is not an offence (the truth is, it is probably as much a disappointment to the therapist as it is to you). But failure to take proper care and treat you with professional respect is.

If this should happen to you, and you feel it is as a result of behaviour which you regard as either incompetent or unethical, you could take the following actions:

- If you feel the therapist was doing his or her best to help – and obviously most try to – but simply wasn't good enough, it might be as well, for the safety of future patients as much as for the therapist's sake, to talk the problem over with him or her first. They may be oblivious of their shortcomings and be not only grateful for your constructive honesty but see a way to make amends and help you further. But if the situation is more serious than this, then you have no option but either to turn your back on the whole episode or to take action. If you decide to take further action the courses open to you are:

- Report them to their professional association or society if they have one. Don't expect this to lead to dramatic changes, however. Because unconventional medicine still belongs to an unestablished, and even sometimes anti-establishment, subculture – it has been called 'the folk medicine of the masses' – it still exists in many countries in a sort of unregulated limbo world in which pretty well anything goes and there are few official controls. This can have its advantages, of course: the better and more original practitioners can experiment and change direction at will in a way they would not be allowed to if they were tied up by rules and regulations as doctors are. But it also means there is little or no professional comeback if they don't behave in a way you like or think they should. Even if they belong to a professional organization – and, in Britain at least, no practitioner who is not medically trained has to belong to any organization – those organizations have little or no real power to do anything to a member who breaks the rules. In Britain, if they expel someone that person is still free to practise under existing common law provided they don't break any civil or criminal law.

● Tell anyone and everyone you come across about your experience, especially the person who recommended the therapist (if this applies), and tell the therapist himself or herself that you are doing so (but make sure you are telling the truth: deliberately spreading lies which damage someone's reputation and livelihood is a criminal offence). Practitioners who get themselves a bad reputation are quickly out of business – and rightly so – and therefore, to that extent at least, they are under pressure to behave professionally, and they know it. Ultimately that is your only guarantee. But it is also the best guarantee.

● In the very worst case, which is always possible, though rare, you can resort to the civil or criminal law – that is, you can sue or bring a charge for assault, either through a lawyer or by going directly to the police. Alternatively, citizens' rights or advice bureaux may be able to help.

Summary

The reality is that, although the opportunity is there, resulting in the occasional tabloid newspaper headline, there are few real crooks or charlatans in natural therapy. Despite the myth, there is still little real money in it unless the therapist is very busy – and if he or she is, the chances are high that it is because he or she is good. In fact, you are just as likely to find bad practitioners in conventional medicine and among the ranks of the so-called 'qualified' as among those who work quietly alone at home with no formal training at all. No one can know everything and no one qualified in anything, including medicine, has to get 100 per cent in their exams to be able to practise. Perfection is an ideal, not a reality, and to err is human.

It is very much for this reason that taking control of your own health is perhaps the single most important lesson underlying the series of books of which this is part. For taking control means taking responsibility for the choices you make, and taking responsibility for choices is, we now know, one of the most significant factors in successful treatment, whether by yourself or through the intermediate services of a therapist.

No one but you can decide on a practitioner and no one but you should decide if that practitioner is any good or not, whether he or she is a conventional doctor or a natural therapist or both. You will know very easily, and probably very quickly, if they are any good by the way you feel about them and their therapy, and by whether or not you get any better.

If you are not happy about them or your progress the decision is yours whether to stay or move on – and continue moving until you find the right therapist for you. But do not despair if you don't find the right person first time, and above all never give up hope. There is almost bound to be the right person for you somewhere, and your determination to get well is the best resource you have for finding them.

Above all, bear in mind that many people who have taken this route before you have not only been helped beyond their most optimistic dreams but have also found a close and trusted helper whom they, and their family, can always turn to in times of trouble – and who may even become a friend for life.

APPENDIX A

Useful organizations

The following listing of organizations is for information only and does not imply any endorsement, nor do the organizations listed necessarily agree with the views expressed in this book.

INTERNATIONAL

International Federation of Practitioners of Natural Therapeutics
46 Pulens Crescent
Sheet
Petersfield
Hampshire GU31 4DH, UK.
Tel 0730 266790
Fax 0730 260058

International Foundation for Bowel Dysfunction
PO Box 17864
Milwaukee
Wisconsin 53217, USA.
Tel 414 964 1799

AUSTRALASIA

Acupuncture Ethics and Standards Organization
PO Box 84
Merrylands
New South Wales 2160
Australia.

Australian Natural Therapists Association
PO Box 308
Melrose Park
South Australia 5039.
Tel 8297 9533
Fax 8297 0003

Australian Traditional Medicine Society
PO Box 442 *or*
Suite 3, First Floor
120 Blaxland Road
Ryde
New South Wales 2112
Australia.
Tel 2808 2825
Fax 2809 7570

International Federation of Aromatherapists
35 Bydown Street
Neutral Bay
New South Wales 2089
Australia.

New Zealand Natural Health
Practitioners Accreditation
Board
PO Box 37-491
Auckland, New Zealand.
Tel 9 625 9966
*Supported by 15 therapy
organizations.*

New Zealand Register of
Acupuncturists
PO Box 9950
Wellington 1
New Zealand.

NORTH AMERICA

American Academy of Medical
Preventics
6151 West Century Boulevard,
Suite 1114
Los Angeles
California 90045, USA.
Tel 213 645 5350

American Aromatherapy
Association
PO Box 3609
Culver City
California 90231, USA.

American Association of
Acupuncture and Oriental
Medicine
National Acupuncture
Headquarters
1424 16th Street NW,
Suite 501
Washington DC 200 36, USA.

American Association of
Naturopathic Physicians
2800 East Madison Street
Suite 200
Seattle
Washington 98112, USA
or
PO Box 20386
Seattle
Washington 98102, USA.
Tel 206 323 7610
Fax 206 323 7612

American Holistic Medical
Association
4101 Lake Boone Trail, Suite 201
Raleigh
North Carolina 27607, USA.
Tel 919 787 5146
Fax 919 787 4916

American Gastroenterological
Association Foundation
Suite 914
7910 Woodmount Avenue
Bethesda
Maryland 20814, USA.

B.K.S. Iyengar Yoga National
Association of the United States
8223 West Third Street
Los Angeles
California 90038, USA.

Canadian Holistic Medical
Association
700 Bay Street
PO Box 101, Suite 604
Toronto
Ontario M5G 1Z6, Canada.
Tel 416 599 0447

North American Society of Homoeopaths
4712 Aldrich Avenue
Minneapolis 55409, USA.

SOUTHERN AFRICA

South African Homoeopaths, Chiropractors & Allied Professions Board
PO Box 17055
0027 Groenkloof
South Africa
Tel 2712 466 455

UNITED KINGDOM

British Association for Counselling
37a Sheep Street
Rugby
Warwickshire CV21 3BY.
Tel 01788 578328

British Association of Psychotherapists
37 Mapesbury Road
London NW2 4HJ.
Tel 0181 452 9823
Fax 0181 452 5182

British Complementary Medicine Association
St Charles Hospital
Exmoor Street
London W10 6DZ.
Tel 0181 964 1205
Fax 0181 964 1207

British Digestive Foundation
3 St Andrew's Place
London NW1 4LB.
Tel 0171 487 5332

British Homoeopathic Association
27a Devonshire Street
London W1N 1RJ.
Tel 0171 935 2163
Medically qualified homoeopaths only

British Medical Acupuncture Society
Newton House
Newton Lane
Lower Whitley
Warrington, Cheshire WA4 4JA.
Tel 01925 730727

British Society for Medical and Dental Hypnosis
42 Links Road
Ashtead
Surrey KT21 2HJ.
Tel 01372 273522

British Society for Nutritional Medicine
Stone House
9 Weymouth Street
London W1N 3FF.
Tel 0171 436 8532

Council for Complementary & Alternative Medicine
179 Gloucester Place
London NW1 6DX.
Tel 0171 724 9103
Fax 0171 724 5330

Institute for Complementary Medicine
PO Box 194
London SE16 1QZ.
Tel 0171 237 5165
Fax 0171 237 5175

British Holistic Medical Association
179 Gloucester Place
London NW1 6DX.
Tel 0171 262 5299

Health Education Authority
Hamilton House
Mabledon Place
London WC1H 9TX.
Tel 0171 383 3833
Fax 0171 387 0550

National Institute of Medical Herbalists
56 Longbrook Street
Exeter
Devon EX4 6AH.
Tel 01392 426022
Fax 01392 498963

Research Council for Complementary Medicine
60 Great Ormond Street
London WC1N 3JF.
Tel 0171 833 8897

Yoga Biomedical Trust
PO Box 140
Cambridge CB4 3SY.
Tel 01223 67301

Yoga for Health Foundation
Ickwell Bury
Biggleswade
Bedfordshire SG18 9EF
Tel 01767 627271

Self-help group
Christine Dancey
IBS Network
c/o Wells Park Health Project
1a Wells Park Road
Sydenham,
London SE26 6JE.
Tel 0181 291 3332

APPENDIX B

Useful further reading

Acupuncture, George Lewith (Thorsons, London, 1982)

Complementary Medicine and Disability: Alternatives for People with Disabling Conditions, Andrew Vickers (Chapman & Hall, UK, 1993)

The Complete Yoga Course, Howard Kent (Headline Press, UK, 1993)

Coping Successfully with Your Irritable Bowel, R. Nicol (Sheldon Press, UK, 1989)

Eating Right for a Bad Gut: The Complete Nutritional Guide, James Scala (Hal/Dutton, USA, 1990)

Gastrointestinal Health: A Self-help Nutritional Program, Steven Peikin (HarperCollins, USA, 1992)

Gentle Medicine: Thorsons Concise Encyclopaedia of Natural Health, Angela Smyth (Thorsons, UK, 1994)

Holistic Living, Dr Patrick Pietroni (Dent, UK, 1986)

IBS Handbook: Learning to Live with Irritable Bowel Syndrome, Gerard Guillory (MTA Publishing, USA, 1989)

Irritable Bowel and Diverticulosis: A Self-help Plan (Thorsons, UK, 1990)

Irritable Bowel Syndrome, ed Nicholas Read (Saunders, USA, 1985)

The Irritable Bowel Syndrome: A Practical Guide, Dr Geoff Watts (Cedar Press, UK, 1990)

Overcoming IBS: Practical Help in Coping with Irritable Bowel Syndrome, Christine Dancey and Susan Blackhouse (Robinson, UK, 1993)

Reader's Digest Family Guide to Alternative Medicine, ed Dr Patrick Pietroni (Reader's Digest Association, UK, 1991)

Relief from Irritable Bowel Syndrome, Elaine Shimberg (Evans, USA, 1988)

The Wellness Book of IBS: How to Achieve Relief from Irritable Bowel Syndrome, Deralee Scanlon (St Martin's Press, USA, 1991)

Index